Trauma, Pedagogy, and the College Mental Health Crisis

W0018690

Trauma, Pedagogy, and the College Mental Health Crisis argues that psychoanalytic theory and practice offer a solution to the large increase in students seeking mental health services.

Robert Samuels returns to the roots of psychoanalysis, drawing from Freud's and Lacan's conceptions of hysteria and narcissism. This book examines the idea that the repression of psychoanalysis has resulted in a situation where students are being misdiagnosed and mistreated as the underlying structures shaping narcissism and hysteria are misrecognized. Samuels suggests that the more people are trained to focus on their own thoughts and feelings, the more they take on self-destructive thoughts and behaviors in a neurotic way and that psychoanalysis offers a solution.

Trauma, Pedagogy, and the College Mental Health Crisis will be of interest to psychoanalysts in practice and in training, as well as mental health professionals working with adolescents and professionals working in higher education. It will also be relevant to readers interested in adolescent mental health, higher education, parenting, and politics.

Robert Samuels holds doctorates in psychoanalysis and English and teaches advanced writing at the University of California, Santa Barbara. He is the author of 25 books, including *Political Pathologies from The Sopranos to Succession: Prestige TV and the Contradictions of the "Liberal" Class* and *Teaching Writing, Rhetoric, and Reason at the Globalizing University* (both Routledge).

Trauma, Pedagogy, and the College Mental Health Crisis

Hysteria, Narcissism, and the Repression of Psychoanalysis

Robert Samuels

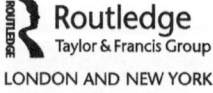

Routledge
Taylor & Francis Group

LONDON AND NEW YORK

Designed cover image: Getty | jacoblund

First published 2025
by Routledge
4 Park Square, Milton Park, Abingdon, Oxon OX14 4RN

and by Routledge
605 Third Avenue, New York, NY 10158

Routledge is an imprint of the Taylor & Francis Group, an informa business

British Library Cataloguing-in-Publication Data
A catalogue record for this book is available from the British Library

ISBN: 978-1-032-89993-0 (hbk)
ISBN: 978-1-032-89992-3 (pbk)
ISBN: 978-1-003-54566-8 (ebk)

DOI: 10.4324/9781003545668

Typeset in Times New Roman
by Apex CoVantage, LLC

Contents

Chapter 1

Introduction

I started off writing a book about the focus on trauma in teaching college writing, but I soon realized that it was impossible to examine this issue without looking at the broader social implications. I also wanted to address what has been called the college mental health crisis and the way that psychoanalysis has been repressed in these discussions.[1] My central thesis is that the misunderstanding of hysteria and narcissism has helped to create a situation where psychological suffering is accommodated and reinforced by narcissistic individuals and institutions. Unfortunately, few people understand Freud's notions of hysteria and narcissism, and instead, what we are seeing is the drugging of discontent and the application of destructive models of therapy. By carefully reading recent works from psychology, education theory, sociology, and the new brain sciences, I hope to offer an effective alternative to the current manufactured crisis.

Defining Trauma

One of the first problems we encounter is that it is unclear how to define trauma and how to treat it and other forms of psychological suffering.[2] We shall see that due to an ever-expanded definition of trauma, the difference between real and imagined trauma has often been lost.[3] In fact, many theorists, educators, and psychologists argue that almost everyone has been traumatized, and so what we need to do is respond with empathy and accommodation to all individual claims, but the question arises: what happens to education, science, and liberal democracy when the focus is placed on the suffering subject?[4]

On the most basic level, the ideals of neutrality, objectivity, and equality are being undermined by an emphasis on emotion, empathy, and mind control. Instead of recognizing the importance and meaning of transference, drives, the primary processes, the unconscious, and free association, a pre-psychoanalytic understanding of "human nature" is applied.[5] For instance, we find a repression of Freud's central notion that people are unaware of how they use the expression of suffering in order to manipulate others and their own identities.[6] Likewise, the desire to see oneself as good and virtuous pushes parents, therapists, and educators to hide their own hostility, guilt, and shame behind acts of demonstrated goodness.[7] Although it appears that there is

DOI: 10.4324/9781003545668-1

nothing wrong with being altruistic, the problem is that when someone is acting to protect their own positive self-image, they may repress the negative effects of their actions as they seek to escape any feelings of guilt and shame. Moreover, when institutions and teachers take on the role of nurturing parents, their displays of care can act to reinforce destructive unconscious pathologies.[8]

Of course, there is still a need to affirm that people really do suffer from traumatic events, but when our definition of trauma becomes over-generalized, it becomes difficult to distinguish between real and imagined experiences. As is well-known, Freud started off thinking that all of his female patients were sexually abused by their fathers, but he soon realized that some of them only imagined their abuse.[9] He then had to determine why someone would invent their own trauma and suffering. His fundamental response was that by taking on the identity of being a victim, one can remove oneself from criticism, responsibility, and the sacrifices required by society.[10] He also affirmed that male and female hysterics usually are not consciously aware of what they are doing, and the distinction between the mind and the body is undermined. By using their bodies to communicate in an indirect way, hysterics are able to influence people on the level of emotions and not through power or reason.[11]

In our current culture, it is common for people to seek out a mental health diagnosis in order to gain a sense of identity and to justify their lives and actions.[12] This process is enabled by institutions that provide diagnostic categories and related methods of care. Thus, one reason why we are experiencing a mental health crisis at college campuses is that students are seeking out diagnostic identities, and the institutions are responding by reinforcing these desires.[13] Meanwhile, political groups are often shaped by the affirmation of a victim identity and a group's victim identification.[14] Although it is important to stress that there are individuals and groups who have been abused and exploited, psychoanalysis pushes us to ask how people use their victim status to affect others and rewrite their own histories and identities.

Instead of using core psychoanalytic concepts to examine hysteria and narcissism, we find educators, therapists, and parents tending to reinforce destructive psychopathologies in an effort to feel good about themselves. We also see a turn to practices like Cognitive Behavioral Therapy (CBT) as a quick fix to human suffering and discontent, but this method relies on a return to mental suggestion and other modes of mind control.[15] While Freud developed psychoanalysis by rejecting his initial use of hypnosis, practitioners of CBT show little understanding of transference, the unconscious, the primary processes, drives, and free association.[16] Thus, rather than reducing someone's dependence on idealized others (transference), these therapists simply rewrite someone's thinking by replacing negative ideas with positive ones. CBT, then, is a method of forced adaptation and conformity, which enables people with power to repress the true causes of discontent.[17]

For Freud, the ultimate driving force behind human misery is the unresolvable conflict between society and the individual.[18] Although this divide can never be fully healed, what we discover through free association is the need for people to confront the truth of how this conflict affects them. The irony of our current situation is that while the scientific and therapeutic value of psychoanalysis has been called into question, the brain sciences have taken on the role of explaining human subjectivity and culture, and yet these new sciences are often pseudo-sciences shaped by bad definitions and forced conclusions.[19] In an effort to erase the importance of subjectivity, history, culture, and education, biological determinism is used to remove personal and social responsibility in order to blame everything on inherited mental programs passed on by our genes.[20] The ultimate result of this perspective is to see medication as the only solution to human suffering.[21] We are thus over-diagnosed, over-medicated, and overly catered to as we seek to repress the true causes of our discontent.

Book Outline

In Chapter 2, I examine the possible connection between the increase in reported student anxiety and depression in college and the habitual use of smartphones and social media. As Jean Twenge argues in her *Why Today's Super-Connected Kids Are Growing Up Less Rebellious, More Tolerant, Less Happy – and Completely Unprepared for Adulthood – and What That Means for the Rest of Us*, we can match the rise in young adult mental suffering with their excessive use of these new technologies, but what needs to be explored is how does this addiction to Web-based media produce the symptoms of depression and anxiety?[22] As I will argue, students often present hysterical symptoms that are catered to by narcissistic parents, therapists, and educators, and so it is vital to comprehend how to respond to these complaints.

Chapter 3 looks at the history and current use of what is now called trauma-informed pedagogy in order to articulate the main motivations and effects of this educational strategy.[23] Although my focus is on the field of college writing, much of the discussion can be applied to many other disciplines and aspects of contemporary society. The main argument is that a misguided understanding of trauma and therapy threatens to undermine higher education in particular and modern reason in general from within. Through a careful reading of Michelle Day's dissertation "Wounds and Writing: Building Trauma-Informed Approaches to Writing Pedagogy," I expose the roots of a destructive educational ideology.[24]

Chapter 4 analyzes how politics has helped to shape the ways we think about student mental health, trauma, and the role of higher education in responding to the mental suffering of students. In examining Greg Lukianoff's and Jonathan Haidt's *The Coddling of the American Mind*, we discover that social perceptions of student mental health issues have been affected by a center-Right ideology combining together conservative morality with a backlash against Left-wing politics and educational activism.[25] Furthermore, a commonly proposed solution, CBT, represents the repression of psychoanalysis and a new form of hypnotic mind control. Through the combination of premodern moralism and libertarian capitalism, a false form of liberalism is presented, and one of the results is that hysteria and narcissism continue to be reinforced.

Chapter 5 looks at the conservative response to the college mental health crisis and the call to use CBT to change these students' hearts and minds. In order to further examine the conflicting conceptions of student suffering and educational therapy, I turn to Farhad Dalal's *CBT: The Cognitive Behavioural Tsunami*, which offers an insightful analysis of how the study of mental health treatment is often manipulated inside and outside of higher education.[26] In relating CBT to Freud's early use of hypnosis and suggestion, I show why Freud moved to analytic neutrality and free association as a more effective way of dealing with mental health issues.

Chapter 6 looks at several of the ways that psychoanalysis is being undermined from within psychoanalysis through the formation of a narcissistic mode of therapy. We shall see that by emphasizing trauma and misrepresenting hysteria and narcissism, a false model of analysis is presented. While the writers of the book *A New Vision of Psychoanalytic Theory, Practice and Supervision* believe that they are still doing psychoanalysis, it should be evident that their theories and practices have little to do with what Freud invented.[27] In fact, I will argue that their beliefs undermine our ability to fix the college mental health crisis because they fail to understand why and how humans use suffering to gain a sense of identity while they unconsciously manipulate others on an emotional level. Moreover, the kind of therapy they present matches many of the educational responses to trauma that we are currently encountering. In turning to Abigail Shrier's *Bad Therapy,* I will examine some of the ways the confusion of parenting with therapy has shaped contemporary college students.[28]

To further examine the college mental health crisis, Chapter 7 turns to Matthew Bowker's *A Dangerous Place to Be: Identity, Conflict, and Trauma in Higher Education*, which makes the provocative argument that many of the causes for student suffering and ineffective institutional responses stem from the idea that people are treating universities as substitute families.[29] Moreover, Bowker believes that the type of family dynamics being projected onto these schools derives from a fundamental fear that parents have regarding their children's desires and impulses.

The final chapter outlines some of the actions that universities and colleges can employ to fix the college mental health crisis. One of the major things I stress is the need to define and defend the principles of academic culture, which include truth, honesty, impartiality, empiricism, and universality. In looking at Freud's theory of the realty principle, I emphasize the need to make the unbiased search for the truth of reality to be the core mission of the institutions of higher education.[30] I also advocate for limiting the use of technology in the classroom as a way of helping to break students' addiction to new media devices. It is also important to stop seeing universities as places to promote politics and therapy, and this requires reducing the amount of funds spent on student services and other non-educational activities. The overall message of this book is that the repression of psychoanalysis has resulted in a situation where students are being misdiagnosed and mistreated as the underlying structures shaping narcissism and hysteria are misrecognized.

Notes

1   Kadison, Richard, and Theresa Foy DiGeronimo. *College of the Overwhelmed: The Campus Mental Health Crisis and What to Do about It.* Vol. 6. San Francisco, CA: Jossey-Bass, 2004.
2   Weathers, Frank W., and Terence M. Keane. "The criterion a problem revisited: Controversies and challenges in defining and measuring psychological trauma." *Journal of Traumatic Stress* 20.2 (2007): 107–121.

3 Gradus, Jaimie L., and Sandro Galea. "Reconsidering the definition of trauma." *The Lancet Psychiatry* 9.8 (2022): 608–609.

4 Thompson, Lee, Michael Hill, and Gary Shaw. "Defining major trauma: A literature review." *British Paramedic Journal* 4.1 (2019): 22–30.

5 Samuels, Robert. *The Psychoanalytic Understanding of Consciousness, Free Will, Language, and Reason: What Makes Us Human?* Routledge, 2023.

6 Fishbain, David A., et al. "Secondary gain concept: A review of the scientific evidence." *The Clinical Journal of Pain* 11.1 (1995): 6–21.

7 Samuels, Robert. "(Liberal) narcissism." *Routledge Handbook of Psychoanalytic Political Theory*. Routledge, 2019, 151–161.

8 Ahmadi, Vahid, Abbas Nasrolahi, and Sareh Mirshekar. "Examining the simple and multiple relationship of parenting styles and early life trauma with narcissistic personality in university students." *Archives of Advances in Biosciences* 6.1 (2015).

9 Israëls, Han, and Morton Schatzman. "The seduction theory." *History of Psychiatry* 4.13 (1993): 23–59.

10 Freud, Sigmund. *Dora: An Analysis of a Case of Hysteria*. Simon and Schuster, 1997.

11 Micale, Mark S. "Hysteria and its historiography: A review of past and present writings (I)." *History of Science* 27.3 (1989): 223–261.

12 O'Connor, Cliodhna, et al. "How does psychiatric diagnosis affect young people's self-concept and social identity? A systematic review and synthesis of the qualitative literature." *Social Science & Medicine* 212 (2018): 94–119.

13 Wiley, Adrianna. *A Thorn by Any Other Name: Exploring University Students' Constructs of Mental Health and the Creation of Positive Identity*. Diss. University of Guelph, 2022.

14 Samuels, Robert, and Robert Samuels. "Pathos, Hysteria, and the left." *Zizek and the Rhetorical Unconscious: Global Politics, Philosophy, and Subjectivity*. Springer, 2020, 33–47.

15 Yapko, Michael. "Suggesting mindfulness: Awakening the hypnotist within." *Australian Journal of Clinical Hypnotherapy and Hypnosis* 34.2 (2012): 5–19.

16 Aron, Lewis. "From hypnotic suggestion to free association: Freud as a psychotherapist, circa 1892–1893." *Contemporary Psychoanalysis* 32.1 (1996): 99–114.

17 Longmore, Richard J., and Michael Worrell. "Do we need to challenge thoughts in cognitive behavior therapy?" *Clinical Psychology Review* 27.2 (2007): 173–187.

18 Freud, Sigmund. *Civilization and Its Discontents*. Broadview Press, 2015.

19 Samuels, Robert. *Psychoanalyzing the Politics of the New Brain Sciences*. Springer, 2017.

20 Lewontin, Richard C., Steven Rose, and Leon J. Kamin. *Not in Our Genes*. New York: Pantheon Books, 1984.

21 Samuels, Robert, and Robert Samuels. "Drugging discontent: Psychoanalysis, drives, and the governmental university medical pharmaceutical complex (GUMP)." *Psychoanalyzing the Politics of the New Brain Sciences*. Springer, 2017, 115–136.

22 Twenge, Jean M. *iGen: Why Today's Super-Connected Kids Are Growing Up Less Rebellious, More Tolerant, Less Happy – and Completely Unprepared for Adulthood – and What That Means for the Rest of Us*. Simon and Schuster, 2017.

23 Harrison, Neil, Jacqueline Burke, and Ivan Clarke. "Risky teaching: Developing a trauma-informed pedagogy for higher education." *Teaching in Higher Education* 28.1 (2023): 180–194.

24 Day Michelle. *Wounds and Writing: Building Trauma-Informed Approaches to Writing Pedagogy*. PhD dissertation. University of Louisville, 2019.

25 Lukianoff, Greg, and Jonathan Haidt. *The Coddling of the American Mind: How Good Intentions and Bad Ideas Are Setting Up a Generation for Failure*. Penguin, 2019.

26 Dalal, Farhad. *CBT: The Cognitive Behavioural Tsunami: Managerialism, Politics and the Corruptions of Science*. Routledge, 2018.

27 Brothers, Doris, and Jon Sletvold. *A New Vision of Psychoanalytic Theory, Practice and Supervision: Talking Bodies*. Routledge, 2023.

28 Shrier, Abigail. *Bad Therapy: Why the Kids Aren't Growing Up*. Swift Press, 2024.
29 Bowker, Matthew H., and David P. Levine. *A Dangerous Place to Be: Identity, Conflict, and Trauma in Higher Education*. Routledge, 2018.
30 Samuels, Robert, and Robert Samuels. "Science and the reality principle." *Freud for the Twenty-First Century: The Science of Everyday Life*. Springer, 2019, 5–16.

Chapter 2

Misdiagnosing Students

One possible cause for the increase in reported student anxiety and depression on college campuses could be the habitual use of smartphones and social media. As Jean Twenge argues in her *Why Today's Super-Connected Kids Are Growing Up Less Rebellious, More Tolerant, Less Happy – and Completely Unprepared for Adulthood – and What That Means for the Rest of Us*, we can match the rise in young adult mental suffering with their excessive use of these new technologies, but what needs to be explored is how does this addiction to Web-based media produce the symptoms of depression and anxiety?[1] As I will argue, students often present hysterical symptoms that are catered to by narcissistic parents, therapists, and educators, and so it is vital to comprehend how to respond to these complaints.

Changing Life Patterns

Twenge posits that one reason why students appear to be suffering so much in college is that they are not prepared to be on their own: "compared to their predecessors, iGen teens are less likely to go out without their parents, date, have sex, drive, work, or drink alcohol" (51). In other words, before many of these young adults show up on campus, they have grown up in a world where they mostly stay alone at home, and they may not be going out or experimenting with drugs and sex because they are more comfortable experiencing things online.[2] Moreover, their parents are also supportive of this isolation since they are afraid to let their children go outside and interact with unknown people.[3] New media technologies, then, serve to occupy isolated young adults and also isolate them even more.

For Twenge, the most current generation of children and young adults, which she calls the iGeneration, has a very different upbringing than previous generations since they have never known a time without smartphones and social media: "iGen'ers are strikingly less likely to experience these once nearly universal adolescent milestones, those breathtaking first experiences of independence from your parents that leave you feeling, for the first time, that you're an adult" (51). From this perspective, what helps cause college student anxiety and depression is that these young people are unprepared to be on their own, and they have little experience with social relationships, drugs, sex, and alcohol.[4] Thus, once they arrive at

DOI: 10.4324/9781003545668-2

higher education institutions, they may not know how to act or feel, and they may be unable to control their use of addictive substances.

Instead of merely blaming technology, then, Twenge focuses mainly on changing family dynamics as she demonstrates how young people are not maturing like they once did: "Childhood has lengthened, with teens treated more like children, less independent and more protected by parents than they once were" (53). Due to this extension of childhood and the delay in becoming an adult, these young people remain highly centered on their own selves:

> The cultural shift toward individualism may also play a role: childhood and adolescence are uniquely self-focused stages, so staying in them longer allows more cultivation of the individual self. With fewer children and more time spent with each, each child is noticed and celebrated.
>
> (54)

This focus on the individual child can breed higher rates of narcissism and hysteria because both of these mods of neurosis are based on how people seek the attention and affirmation of others: in the case of narcissism, one wants to have the good self recognized, and, with hysteria, one desires to have one's suffering affirmed.[5] Moreover, when the other does not affirm these desires, the result can be a generation of anxiety, which Freud relates to a fear of lost love coupled with the lack of protection against a threatening external world.[6]

In turning to neuroscience, Twenge insists that these young adults do not have fully developed brains: "Maybe today's teens and young adults have an underdeveloped frontal cortex because they have not been given adult responsibilities" (55). This use of the new brain sciences tells us very little because we still need to know why and how they are not developing. For Twenge, the main culprit appears to be protective parents: "Parents do keep a closer watch over teens these days. More teens say that their parents always know where they are and who they are with when they go out at night" (55). This emphasis on overly protective parents forces us to ask: why are parents acting this way?[7] Is their fear of the external world a product of their own phobias?[8] It is my hypothesis that a combination of harmful psychological ideas combined with a culture of fear has led to young people turning to new media technologies as a drug bent on reducing anxiety and also helping young people find a fixed hysterical identity.[9] To make this argument, I will first turn to Christopher Lasch's *Culture of Narcissism*, which exposes many of the roots of this current dynamic.[10]

Revisiting the Culture of Narcissism

Lasch's 1979 book argues that we have moved from a culture shaped by religion to one influenced by therapy: "The contemporary climate is therapeutic, not religious. People today hunger not for personal salvation, let alone for the restoration of an earlier golden age, but for the feeling, the momentary illusion, of personal well-being, health, and psychic security" (7). According to this theory, instead of individuals today respecting authority and religious morality, they are driven by a personal desire for safety and well-being. Since secularism and capitalism have undermined patriarchy and religion, the classic resolution of the Oedipus complex has been suspended, as people are left on their own in order to gain a sense of identity, meaning, and protection.[11] In this gap left open by the loss of traditional values, roles, and authorities, a set of therapeutic ideas have spread through the culture, and these ideas have reshaped what it means to be a parent, teacher, or leader.[12]

On one level, we can trace what Lasch calls the culture of narcissism to a generalized application of therapy to all aspects of contemporary life: "The new therapies spawned by the human potential movement, according to Peter Marin, teach that 'the individual will is all powerful and totally determines one's fate'; thus they intensify the 'isolation of the self'" (10). The idea here is that focusing on individual agency, psychological theories, and therapeutic practices ended up making people feel even more alone.[13] In other words, therapies dedicated to self-improvement have the perverse effect of undermining the self by isolating individuals from each other while undermining all sources of collective knowledge and mediation: "The atrophy of older traditions of self-help has eroded everyday competence, in one area after another, and has made the individual dependent on the state, the corporation, and other bureaucracies" (10). The paradox of this emphasis on the isolated individual is that one becomes even more dependent on outside experts and alienating institutions.[14]

The reason why the narcissistic focus on the self results in alienation and dependency is that the ideal ego needs to be recognized and verified by others: "Narcissism represents the psychological dimension of this dependence. Notwithstanding his occasional illusions of omnipotence, the narcissist depends on others to validate his self-esteem. He cannot live without an admiring audience" (10). Although most people think that narcissists are simply self-centered, Lasch reveals why they are actually obsessed with what others think about them.[15] As Lacan claims, the narcissist is an other for the Other, which means that in order to see the self as being good and competent, one has to conform to the expectation of others, and this conformity has to be recognized by others in order to be validated.[16]

A key then to understanding what can be called obsessional narcissism is the underlying insecurity that drives the search for recognition, love, and knowledge: "His apparent freedom from family ties and institutional constraints does not free him to stand alone or to glory in his individuality. On the contrary, it contributes to his insecurity, which he can overcome only by seeing his "grandiose self" reflected in the attentions of others, or by attaching himself to those who radiate celebrity, power, and charisma" (10). If the narcissist cannot gain recognition for being good from others, there is always the possibility of identifying with others who have been idealized.[17] Lasch's brilliant analysis, then, anticipates our current obsession with celebrities and the use of social media to have one's self recognized by others.[18]

For Lasch, an effect of this narcissistic culture is that people become easily bored since their drives have been repressed in an effort to conform to social norms: "Today Americans are overcome not by the sense of endless possibility but by the banality of the social order they have erected against it. Having internalized the social restraints by means of which they formerly sought to keep possibility within civilized limits, they feel themselves overwhelmed by an annihilating boredom, like animals whose instincts have withered in captivity" (11). As Freud found in his analysis of obsessive-compulsive neurotics, the desire to be validated by others in order to maintain a positive self-image results in a repression of aggression and the release of sexual and violent drives through the indirect means of fantasy.[19] We shall see that contemporary parents often take on a form of obsessional narcissism, and not only do these adults want to be seen as being ideal parents, but they also want to see their idealized children recognized by others for their goodness.[20]

For Lasch, narcissists have a divided nature since, on a superficial level, they appear to be conforming to the expectations of others, but deep down, they are enraged: "Outwardly bland, submissive, and sociable, they seethe with an inner anger for which a dense, overpopulated, bureaucratic society can devise few legitimate outlets" (11). This notion of underlying anger can be related to Freud's idea that obsessionals must constantly signal their virtue to others because they want to hide their own hostility and resentment from themselves.[21] Since they have internalized an overly strict conscience, they repress their sexual and violent impulses, but these drives continue to return on an unconscious level. The way, then, to further defend against these anti-social urges is to engage in acts of demonstrated repentance, which can take the form of hand washing or virtue signaling.[22] Freud went as far as saying that behind every one of their acts of altruism, one can find an effort to repress anti-social hostility.[23]

Lasch believes that when this type of personality becomes dominant in a society, all traditional forms of authority are eroded: "The growth of bureaucracy creates an intricate network of personal relations, puts a premium on social skills, and makes the unbridled egotism of the American Adam untenable. Yet at the same time it erodes all forms of patriarchal authority and thus weakens the social superego, formerly represented by fathers, teachers, and preachers" (13). Lasch is describing here the transition from a premodern culture to a modern liberal democracy, but instead of ascribing this change to the role played by capitalism in undermining all previous traditions and authorities, he blames the development of a new mode of personality coupled with the dominance of bureaucratic institutions in a mass society.[24] What is unclear here is whether a changing social structure transformed the dominant psychopathology or if a new mode of personality changed the society.[25]

The response to the previously mentioned question is probably that social structures and psychological structures feed off of each other in a dialectical manner so that each one affects the other in a self-reinforcing loop. Thus, Lasch insists that society and subjectivity have both become narcissistic and this results in the formation of a permissive society coupled with a paradoxical increase in super-ego severity:

The decline of institutionalized authority in an ostensibly permissive society does not, however, lead to a "decline of the superego" in individuals. It encourages instead the development of a harsh, punitive superego that derives most of its psychic energy, in the absence of authoritative social prohibitions, from the destructive, aggressive impulses within the id. Unconscious, irrational elements in the superego come to dominate its operation. As authority figures in modern society lose their "credibility," the superego in individuals increasingly derives from the child's primitive fantasies about his parents – fantasies charged with sadistic rage – rather than from internalized ego ideals formed by later experience with loved and respected models of social conduct.

(13)

According to this historical and cultural analysis, when a society moves from a reliance on external authorities to one centered on internalized authority, the conscience is experienced as being harsher and even more punitive.[26] In other words, in a seemingly "liberal" society, the internalized super-ego of the narcissist derives its aggression from repressed drives.[27] Likewise, as traditional authority figures lose their respect and credibility, children perceive their parents through the lens of primitive fantasies full of sadistic violence. Since the super-ego is not idealized by the affirmation of an ego ideal, the criticism and interventions of others are experienced as a violent attack on the self.[28] Thus, the narcissist can only tolerate affirmative responses from the other, and all forms of discipline or judgment are perceived as threats to the fragile self.[29]

One reason, then, why so many of our students may feel that they have been traumatized is that they experience any lack of affirmation as a violent attack; moreover, narcissistic parents, therapists, and teachers may seek to protect these students and affirm their suffering becomes they want to be seen as being good, caring people, but as Lasch and Freud insist, behind these altruistic gestures, there may be the effort to repress anti-social hostility.[30] In fact, I have argued that what we now call center-Left liberalism is shaped by these dynamics of virtue signaling coupled with a culture of violent and sexual fantasies.[31] Therefore, the so-called "liberal media" can be understood as embodying this unconscious process of repressing and projecting anti-social impulses into the safe space of shared cultural fantasies. Moreover, the desire to view violent media representations fuels a culture of fear that results in a generalized form of paranoia.[32] Since narcissists are attracted to the representation of violence, they feed a system that focuses on threatening news and fictional depictions of violence, and then they begin to see the external world as more violent than it actually is.[33] It is, therefore, no wonder that these parents want to keep their children at home – since they are so fearful of the outside world, they focus on protecting their children by isolating them. In turn, the children who have been exposed to the same threatening media culture also desire to remain safe at home – alone on their phones.[34]

Lasch posits that a combination of boredom and fear produces a type of personality that suffers from anxiety and depression: "Plagued by anxiety, depression, vague discontents, a sense of inner emptiness, the 'psychological man' of the twentieth century seeks neither individual self-aggrandizement nor spiritual transcendence but peace of mind, under conditions that increasingly militate against it" (13). Writing in 1979, Lasch anticipated our current mental health issues, so we cannot simply blame our problems on new media technologies. While smartphones and social media may have enhanced these issues, it should be clear that the roots of current college student discontent can be traced back to previous generations.

Returning to Twenge

Instead of examining the narcissism of the parents and the culture, Twenge tends to focus on how children and young adults are experiencing their own lives: "Their parents made childhood a wonderful place with lots of praise, an emphasis on fun, and few responsibilities. No wonder they don't want to grow up" (59). From this perspective, what drives young people's anxiety and depression is that they were brought up in a world where they were always having their narcissistic desires affirmed, which not only undermined traditional authority but also absolved them of any responsibility.[35] In this structure, parents are seen as being both too lax and too controlling: "Even once they get to college, students' parents continue to treat them like children. Parents register their adult children for classes, remind them of deadlines, and wake them up in time for class" (59). In what is now called helicopter parenting, many college students still rely on their parents, and their parents continue to monitor and aid their children, but we need to ask what is driving this combination of surveillance and tolerance.[36] Since these parents are not simply watching over these young adults and doing things for them, but they are also trying to support whatever their children think or feel, we find both an undermining of self-efficacy and a reliance on being affirmed.[37] Moreover, in this dynamic, all responsibility and criticism is removed as the idealized child is being protected from a perceived dangerous world.

Twenge depicts that instead of college students rejecting their parents' over-involvement, they often ask for it: "Thus the generational sweep is complete: never having known another parenting style, iGen doesn't rebel against their parents' overprotection – instead, they embrace it" (60). Twenge goes on to tie this desire to be protected by parents to the call for trigger warnings and safe spaces by contemporary college students: " 'We want you to treat us like children, not adults,' one college student told a startled faculty member. Some suggest that this cocoon mentality is behind recent campus trends such as 'trigger warnings' to alert students that a reading or lecture material might be disturbing and 'safe spaces' where students can go if they are upset by a campus speaker's message" (60). Since these young adults are used to being protected from a threatening world, they expect their colleges to do anything they can to maintain their psychological comfort and safety – and schools often comply.[38]

This desire to remain a child is evident in Twenge's description of a safe space for college students: "One safe space, for example, featured coloring books and videos of frolicking puppies, neatly connecting the idea of safe spaces with that of childhood" (61). In this desire not to grow up and become an adult, we see why it can be hard for colleges and universities to accommodate the demands of students constantly. Since these institutions traditionally play a role in helping children become adults, it is confusing to ask them to treat young adults as children now.

Media Addiction

Like many other people currently studying the college mental health crisis, Twenge shows how the ubiquity of smartphones has radically shaped the psychology of young adults: "Nearly all slept with their phones, putting them under their pillows, on the mattress, or at the very least within arm's reach of the bed. They checked social media websites and watched videos right before they went to bed, and reached for their phones again as soon as they woke up in the morning (they had to – all of them used it as their alarm)" (63). Like many adults, Twenge is rightly concerned by this reliance on smartphones, but what is not fully explored is how a person can become addicted to a media device.[39] In other terms, we have to ask what addictions are and what psychological function they perform.

On the most basic level, psychoanalysis tells us that instead of humans being determined by instincts, they have drives, and these psychological structures combine together a quest for pleasure coupled with a desire to escape from threatening thoughts and feelings.[40] In fact, Freud defines pleasure as the combination of stimulation with a release of mental and physical tension.[41] Moreover, he shows that, unlike other animals, we can become addicted to almost anything, and so we are prone to having our impulses shaped by social and personal experiences.[42] As a defense against anxiety, shame, and guilt, addictions provide a quick and easy escape from our own thoughts and feelings as they also remove us from the threats of external reality and internal conflicts.[43]

We can, therefore, comprehend the smartphone as the perfect drug because it provides immediate access to pleasure and escape, but it is not, for the most part, regulated and de-valorized by society.[44] After all, children see that their parents are also addicted to their phones and other forms of media consumption, so it is hard for these adults to tell their children that they should put away these devices.[45] Moreover, parents often buy smartphones for their children because they think that it will serve as a way of protecting them when they are in danger or in need.[46] These devices, like other media technologies, can also serve busy parents who quickly learn that children can be pacified by their usage. Like a pacifier for babies, smartphones and portable media devices can quickly soothe and occupy children.[47]

By relying on a device for instant pleasure and escape, people lose the ability to comfort themselves or respond effectively to external problems. Furthermore, the dependency on these easily accessible drugs undermines their ability to delay gratification or to work through difficult internal and external issues.[48] Thus, we have fed a culture of addiction, and it is hard to imagine how we can break this dependency. Since people can turn to their phones or computers to directly access pleasure without the need for other people, their usage represents an auto-erotic, anti-social mode of enjoyment, and as many college teachers can attest, it is difficult to get a student to listen in class if they have become habituated to instant gratification.[49]

In terms of producing student anxiety and depression, it is important to separate the different uses of these new media technologies. As Twenge documents, many young adults report that social media feeds their narcissism: "When you go on social media you post a status or you post a picture and all of a sudden you get all those likes, you get all those affirmations from people, and it can be addictive because you have the constant pats on the back that, like, 'You're smart, you're funny, you're attractive,' he says. But, he acknowledges, 'I feel like it's also kind of hollow.'" (72). The flip side of this sense of being validated by others is the anxiety and sadness one feels when one is not being validated.[50]

The use of these devices also feeds the shortening of attention spans and undermines the ability of people to sustain enough attention to read books and other longer forms of text: "Apparently, texting and posting to social media instead of reading books, magazines, and newspapers are not a boon for reading comprehension or academic writing. That might partially be due to the short attention span that new media seem to encourage" (81). Thus, the form of the media helps to shape the minds and desires of the audience, and here we see that a major threat to higher education is a culture of generalized Attention-Deficit Disorder (ADD).[51] In fact, there is some evidence that ADD is really a social symptom and not an actual individual psychopathology.[52] No matter how we see this lack of attention, it represents a major threat to education and student mental health.

Thus, it is hard for contemporary college students to focus on lectures and textbooks because they have become habituated to jumping between different screens and sources of entertainment and information: "One study installed a program on college students' laptops that took a screenshot every five seconds. The researchers found that students switched between tasks every 19 seconds on average. More than 75% of the students' computer windows were open less than one minute. This is a very different experience from sitting and reading a book for hours" (81). Universities and colleges are therefore not only facing a crisis in student mental health, but they are also dealing with a major threat to their ability to educate students effectively: "iGen'ers need textbooks that include interactive activities such as video sharing and questionnaires, but they also need books that are shorter in length and more conversational in their writing style. They are coming to college with much less experience reading, so we have to meet them where they are, while still teaching them what they need to know" (978). As I wrote in *Generation X and the Rise of the Entertainment Subject*, the undermining of education by entertainment really started to take off in the late 1970s as an increasing number of children were left home by working or divorced parents, and these young adults often spent their time watching television, while the entertainment industry started to cater more to their desires.[53] What happens with the iPhone and the laptop computer is that access to entertainment is greatly enhanced.

With easy access to media entertainment, children have dramatically reduced the time they spend with their peers: "The number of teens who get together with their friends every day has been cut in half in just fifteen years, with especially steep declines recently" (88). As Twenge argues, this lost time with peers can function to undermine the basic social skills of these children and young adults: "An hour a day less spent with friends is an hour a day less spent building social skills, negotiating relationships, and navigating emotions" (89). When these young people show up on college campuses, they often have little experience negotiating relationships and dealing with other people's emotions.[54]

Instead of looking at the broader cultural and psychological reasons for this lack of in-person social interaction, Twenge mainly blames smartphones and social media: "The timing of the recent, severe drop in going out and getting together with friends is highly suspicious: it occurred right when smartphones became popular and social media use really took off" (90). While I have no doubt that these technologies have made the problem worse, it is vital to understand the longer history behind this transformation.

We also have to ask why young people would choose their phones over real people and real activities, and the answer to this complicated question returns us to the issues of addictions, narcissism, and anxiety. Since people are guided by the pleasure principle, they are driven to escape displeasure and access pleasure in the easiest ways possible.[55] We are, therefore, prone to addiction because we have a hard time controlling our impulses – especially when they provide instant stimulation. If we use pornography as an example of the pleasure principle, we find that the easy accessibility of stimulation and release undermines the reality principle and the need to delay gratification.[56] Pornography also teaches us that people will accept the replacement of real interaction with a virtual one, and once a culture makes this type of immediate pleasure available, it is hard to contain it.[57] We also know that people who spend a great amount of time consuming pornography find sex with real people to be unsatisfying since pornographic videos and images often present an idealized object of desire.[58]

Like most addictions, what starts out as a process to attain individual pleasure often ends up being self-destructive, and the more that someone feels guilt and shame regarding their anti-social addiction, the more they turn to that addiction to escape their negative feelings, which can only work on a temporary basis.[59] Unfortunately, our understanding of addictions has been hampered by seeing them as a disease and not as a combination of biological, social, and personal forces.[60] Since people think that they are driven by their genes and neurotransmitters, they might not be motivated to make an effort to change or to understand what is really motivating them.

In terms of institutions of higher education, addiction is a constant mental health issue. One reason why it may be even getting worse is that so many students show up to campus without having any experience with drugs, alcohol, and sex, and thus, they are prone to over-indulge because they have never learned how to moderate their desires.[61] Students also freely admit that the only way they can talk to people at a party is if they are so drunk or high that their normal inhibitions go away, yet this raises the question of why they are so inhibited and afraid.[62] One possible reason is that they are used to interacting with others through a screen that provides a safe distance; moreover, they tend to engage with material and people online that reinforce their own thoughts and feelings.[63] When they have to meet someone new, they may fear being rejected, which generates anxiety, and this anxiety can be released through the use of some addictive, intoxicating material.

It is vital to understand how addiction works if we want to improve the mental health of college students, but as we shall see, this effort to come up with better solutions is hindered by the repression of the psychoanalytic understanding of addiction, anxiety, narcissism, and hysteria. Since there is a tendency to rely on the brain sciences to define human mental functioning, what is often lost is the comprehension of unconscious desires, fears, and defense mechanisms.[64] Furthermore, the proposed solutions to these problems often involve an anti-psychoanalytic understanding of therapy, which results in promoting short solutions like medication and Cognitive Behavioral Therapy (CBT).[65]

Twenge's Narcissism

One cause for our lack of understanding of the college mental health crisis is that we tend to rely on superficial correlations derived from self-reported data and shaped by the questionable definition of key terms. In fact, if we look at Twenge's earlier book, *The Narcissism Epidemic: Living in the Age of Entitlement,* written with Keith Campbell, we find that their way of defining narcissism is misleading: "Narcissism is not simply a confident attitude or a healthy feeling of self-worth . . . narcissists are overconfident, not just confident, and – unlike most people high in self-esteem – place little value on emotionally close relationships" (8).[66] Like so many other people, these authors are confusing narcissism with borderline personality disorders, and this confusion undermines their entire work. Since narcissists have a low underlying self-esteem, they try to cover this insecurity by getting others to validate their competence and goodness.[67] In contrast, people suffering from a borderline personality tend to concentrate on their own id-driven impulses as they are prone to addictions and unstable relationships.[68]

Since Twenge and Campbell misunderstand what narcissistic and borderline personalities entail, all of the survey data they collect is tainted. For instance, when they claim that at least one in ten young adults in their twenties suffer from narcissism, we do not know if they are actually counting people with narcissistic or borderline symptoms (7). In terms of college students, this same use of a faulty definition of narcissism pushes them to equate this disorder with materialism: "Undergraduates are more accepting of the current culture but often report feeling tremendous pressure to self-promote and keep up in a materialistic world" (11). Although the narcissistic desire to be recognized by others can result in self-promotion, the drive for material gain is often part of a borderline mentality.[69] Moreover, these authors clearly argue that narcissism is not based on insecurity, which reveals a major misunderstanding (9).

When the most basic diagnostic categories are misrepresented, the suggestions for responding to these psychopathologies also become faulty, as we see in their discussion of parents relating to young narcissists: "In many cases, the suggested cure for narcissistic behavior is 'feeling good about yourself.' After all, the think-ing goes, fourteen-year-old Megan wouldn't post revealing pictures of herself on MySpace if she had higher self-esteem. So parents redouble their efforts, telling Megan she's special, beautiful, and great. This is like suggesting that an obese person would feel much better if she just ate more doughnuts" (14). While I agree that the response to a narcissistic child's demands is not to reinforce them, what is missing in this description of narcissism is that the posting of pictures online may be derived from an insatiable desire to be recognized and validated.[70] What needs to be examined is what is causing this underlying desire.

Twenge and Campbell think that a young adult like Megan suffers from being over-confident, but as their own example shows, the real problem is a lack of inter-nalized self-value: "Megan wants everyone to see just how beautiful and special she is, and it's not because she thinks she is ugly – it's because she thinks she's hot and, perhaps more importantly, because she lives in a narcissistic society where she might garner praise, status, and 'friends' by displaying blatant sexuality" (15). Since narcissists need to get the validation of their ideal ego from others, they are motivated to represent themselves online through pictures and videos, but this mode of self-display not only puts pressure on people to live up to cultural stand-ards of perfection and beauty, but when these images are not "liked," the result is sadness and an increased sense of insecurity.[71] Meanwhile, when one waits to have one's image liked, one can suffer a great deal of anxiety because, as Lacan argues, we are often anxious when we do not know what the other thinks of us.[72]

Twenge and Campbell argue that one of the major causes for the increase in narcissism is the psychological and therapeutic push to raise people's self-esteem: "In fact, narcissism causes almost all of the things that Americans hoped high self-esteem would prevent, including aggression, materialism, lack of caring for oth-ers, and shallow values. In trying to build a society that celebrates high self-esteem, self-expression, and 'loving yourself,' Americans have inadvertently created more narcissists – and a culture that brings out the narcissistic behavior in all of us" (115). According to this theory, the more that we try to raise people's self-esteem, the more narcissistic they become, but this notion is based on only looking at the expression of grandiosity and not the underlying, unconscious self-doubt.[73]

If we look at the origins of narcissism, we can trace it back to the way that caregivers have to motivate babies to control their bodies – especially toilet train-ing.[74] What people get wrong about Freud's theory of the anal stage and its relation to obsessional neurosis is that it is not primarily a question of the miserly child holding onto their feces.[75] Instead, what is set up by this relationship is the child conforming to the parent or caregiver's demand for cleanliness through bodily con-trol. The narcissistic child learns that he or she can gain a positive response to the demanding adult by revealing a mastery of the body.[76] However, underlying this expression of a competent and good self is a sense of shame and insecurity that comes from the failure to live up to the caregiver's demands and expectations. If we do not recognize the importance of this underlying shame and insecurity, then we misunderstand narcissism.

With the advent of social media, this desire to have the good self recognized by others is only enhanced, and as Lacan points out, this focus on presenting an ideal ego to an other creates an imaginary, dual view of the world, and any time someone else is seen as being validated, the self responds with envy and unconscious aggression.[77] Furthermore, for the beauty industry to convince people to buy their products, they have to convince them first that they are lacking, and thus, they are in need of the provided solution. Advertising not only tells people what they need to buy to look and feel good, it also tells them that they are lacking and should be ashamed of their present state.[78]

For Freud, anxiety is often based on a fear of losing the love and protection of caregivers, and thus, one reason why so many contemporary college students are afraid to talk in class is that they are fearful of being judged and criticized, and this fear can be the result of protecting a fragile ego and preventing an encounter with the unknown.[79] In fact, Freud will equate this lack of preparation for a threatening internal or external reality with trauma, and as we shall see, it is this notion of the traumatic cause that is often misunderstood by teachers, parents, and therapists.[80] In claiming that most students today have been traumatized and experience some form of PTSD, what is missing is the distinction between ordinary external and internal threats and the failure to symbolize and work through traumatic events that return in the form of flashbacks and nightmares.[81] For Freud, this kind of return of the unsymbolized trauma represents a failure of anxiety to signal a threat as it presents a disruption of the pleasure principle's ability to release tension through symbolic substitution.

The Problem With Self-Reporting

It is interesting that Twenge and Campbell's 2009 book does not mention PTSD or trauma; instead, the emphasis is on a false understanding of narcissism. In looking at surveys based on self-reported responses, they indicate how Americans report a high level of self-esteem: "Our country's focus on self-admiration has certainly been successful in raising Americans' opinions of themselves. Self-esteem is at an all-time high in most groups, with more than 80% of recent college students scoring higher in general self-esteem than the average 1960s college student" (17). By relying on surveys and self-reported feelings, these social science researchers fail to consider that people may misrepresent how they really feel to others to gain a sense of praise and to make up for an underlying sense of low self-esteem.[82] Furthermore, the reliance on self-reported feelings completely excludes the unconscious because the unconscious is based on self-deception.[83]

Since some school and governmental policies are being shaped by these questionable surveys, we see how the combination of bad definitions and unreliable data undermines our ability to understand and treat mental health issues. What is remarkable is that Twenge co-writes a book in 2009 centered on narcissism and the problem of inflated self-esteem, but in 2019, she looked at the same groups of people and saw them suffering from anxiety and depression. It is as if the repressed content of her earlier work returns, and now she is obsessed with how new technologies and culture reduce people's self-esteem and sense of security. One reason for this major reversal is that in her initial understanding of narcissism, she confused the desperate attempt for external approval with simple grandiosity: "Other common names for narcissism include arrogance, conceit, vanity, grandiosity, and self-centeredness. A narcissist is full of herself, has a big head, is a blowhard, loves the sound of his own voice, or is a legend in her own mind" (24). The reality is that most narcissists are timid and inhibited, and it is only people who have borderline personalities who are able to act directly on their selfish impulses.[84]

By thinking that college students mostly suffer from an inflated sense of self, psychologists, educators, and parents misunderstand that these young adults are really suffering from high levels of insecurity and shame. Moreover, their use of addictive substances and media serves the purpose of trying to escape this shame and inhibition by using pleasure to block self-monitoring. The solutions to student anxiety and addiction, then, are not based on simply raising their self-esteem or by critiquing them for being selfish or addicted; rather, there needs to be a way of addressing the underlying, unconscious causes of their psychopathology.

The New Hysteria

While the initial use of social media by young adults tended to be connected to this narcissistic structure of having the self liked by others, the second wave can be partially traced back to the use of sites like TikTok, which often cater to the presentation of psychological and physical symptoms.[85] In other words, the first use was narcissistic, but the second use was mostly hysterical since the main effect was to have the expression of suffering affirmed and recognized by others.[86] In fact, studies on the increase in reported Tourette-like symptoms directly relate this new prevalence of physical tics to the millions of videos attached to the display and discussion of this disorder.[87] Just as Freud argued that his hysterical patients had physical impairments that made no anatomical sense, we find that many of the people reporting tics also do not follow any known physical explanation.[88] Young people then make themselves sick by copying the symptoms of others, and this affirmation of a diagnosis gives them a sense of identity and allows them to escape criticism and many social obligations. In what Freud called secondary gain, psychological symptoms can be used as excuses, and on college campuses today, we also see an epidemic of students seeking special treatment and accommodation for real and imagined suffering.[89]

Very few people in higher education want to consider the possibility that students may have fake mental and physical illnesses and that some of their claims of being traumatized may be exaggerated and are being used to gain special accommodations.[90] Due to the desire of narcissistic administrators and faculty to look good by not blaming the victim, what we are seeing are narcissistic responses to hysterical complaints. Furthermore, the COVID epidemic made this problem much worse because, during the height of this real health crisis, schools relaxed most of their policies so that they would not harm students who did not attend class or did not do the work on time.[91] These policies may have made sense at the time, but now there is still a desire not to hold students accountable and to accommodate all of their demands for special treatment.

As we shall see in the next chapter, this relation between hysteria and narcissism in higher education has resulted in a belief that since most of our students have been traumatized, we need to turn education into therapy. My main thesis is that due to the repression of psychoanalysis, college students are being misdiagnosed and mistreated. Moreover, the focus on students as traumatized victims is subverted to the basic principles and ideals of higher education. Rather than teaching these young adults to use reason in order to separate fact from fiction, teachers acting as therapists are catering to hysterical symptoms from a narcissistic position.

Notes

1 Twenge, Jean M. *iGen: Why Today's Super-Connected Kids Are Growing Up Less Rebellious, More Tolerant, Less Happy – and Completely Unprepared for Adulthood – and What That Means for the Rest of Us*. Simon and Schuster, 2017.
2 Ruiz-Casares, Mónica. "'When it's just me at home, it hits me that I'm completely alone': An online survey of adolescents in self-care." *Loneliness Updated*. Routledge, 2013, 154–172.
3 Nelson, Margaret K. *Parenting Out of Control: Anxious Parents in Uncertain Times*. NYU Press, 2010.
4 Marcantonio, Tiffany L., and Kristen N. Jozkowski. "Do college students feel confident to consent to sex after consuming alcohol?" *Journal of American College Health* 71.5 (2023): 1604–1611.
5 Samuels, Robert. *Psychoanalyzing the Left and Right after Donald Trump: Conservatism, Liberalism, and Neoliberal Populisms*. Springer, 2016.
6 Freud, Sigmund, James Strachey, and Alix Strachey. *Inhibitions, Symptoms and Anxiety*. New York: Norton, 1977.
7 Spokas, Megan, and Richard G. Heimberg. "Overprotective parenting, social anxiety, and external locus of control: Cross-sectional and longitudinal relationships." *Cognitive Therapy and Research* 33 (2009): 543–551.
8 Clarke, Kiri, Peter Cooper, and Cathy Creswell. "The parental overprotection scale: Associations with child and parental anxiety." *Journal of Affective Disorders* 151.2 (2013): 618–624.
9 Matar Boumosleh, Jocelyne, and Doris Jaalouk. "Depression, anxiety, and smartphone addiction in university students: A cross sectional study." *PLoS ONE* 12.8 (2017): e0182239.
10 Lasch, Christopher. *The Culture of Narcissism: American Life in an Age of Diminishing Expectations*. New York: Norton, 1979.
11 Fromm, Erich. "The escape from freedom." *An Introduction to Theories of Personality*. Psychology Press, 2014, 121–135.
12 Madsen, Ole Jacob. "Therapeutic cultures: Historical perspectives." *The Routledge International Handbook of Global Therapeutic Cultures*. Routledge, 2020, 14–24.
13 De Vos, Jan, and Jan De Vos. "Therapeutic culture and its discontents: Christopher Lasch's critique of post-war psychologization." *Psychologization and the Subject of Late Modernity* (2013): 73–97.
14 Foster, Roger. "Therapeutic culture, authenticity and neo-liberalism." *History of the Human Sciences* 29.1 (2016): 99–116.

15 Frosh, Stephen, and Stephen Frosh. "Narcissism." *Identity Crisis: Modernity, Psychoanalysis and the Self.* London: Macmillan, 1991, 63–94.
16 Muller, John P. "Ego and subject in Lacan." *Psychoanalytic Review* 69.2 (1982): 234.
17 Freud, Sigmund. *On Narcissism: An Introduction.* Read Books Ltd, 2014.
18 Fox, Claire. "Narcissism and identity." *From Self to Selfie: A Critique of Contemporary Forms of Alienation.* London: Springer, 2019, 167–192.
19 Freud, Sigmund. "Predisposition to the obsessional neurosis." *The Psychoanalytic Review (1913–1957)* 21 (1934): 347.
20 Elkind, David. "Instrumental narcissism in parents." *Bulletin of the Menninger Clinic* 55.3 (1991): 299.
21 Pearson, Judith. "Mirrors of rage: The devaluing narcissistic patient." *Disorders of the Self.* Routledge, 2013, 299–311.
22 Samuels, Robert. *Political Pathologies from the Sopranos to Succession: Prestige TV and the Contradictions of the "Liberal" Class.* Routledge, 2023.
23 Wertz, Frederick. "Freud's case of the rat man revisited: An existential-phenomenological and socio-historical analysis." *Journal of Phenomenological Psychology* 34.1 (2003): 47–78.
24 Marx, Karl, and Friedrich Engels. "The communist manifesto." *Ideals and Ideologies.* Routledge, 2019, 243–255.
25 Samuels, Robert. *The Psychopathology of Political Ideologies.* Routledge, 2021.
26 Freud, Sigmund. "The ego and the id (1923)." *Tacd Journal* 17.1 (1989): 5–22.
27 Žižek, Slavoj. "The vagaries of the superego." *Elementa. Intersections between Philosophy, Epistemology and Empirical Perspectives* 1.1–2 (2022): 13–31.
28 Jesus, Sofia. "Freedom and anxiety: A psychoanalytic exploration of the super-ego in the postmodern era." *Trends in Psychology* (2023): 1–20.
29 Cratsley, Kelso. "Revisiting Freud and Kohut on narcissism." *Theory & Psychology* 26.3 (2016): 333–359.
30 McWilliams, Nancy. "The psychology of the altruist." *Psychoanalytic Psychology* 1.3 (1984): 193.
31 Samuels, Robert. *Political Pathologies from the Sopranos to Succession: Prestige TV and the Contradictions of the "Liberal" Class.* Routledge, 2023.
32 Furedi, Frank. "The only thing we have to fear is the 'culture of fear' itself." *American Journal of Sociology* 32.2 (2007): 231–234.
33 Furedi, Frank. *How Fear Works: Culture of Fear in the Twenty-First Century.* Bloomsbury Publishing, 2018.
34 Cantor, Joanne, and Karyn Riddle. "Media and fear in children and adolescents." *Media Violence and Children* (2003): 185–203.
35 Rappoport, Alan. "Co-narcissism: How we accommodate to narcissistic parents." *The Therapist* 1 (2005): 1–8.
36 Schiffrin, Holly H., et al. "Helping or hovering? The effects of helicopter parenting on college students' well-being." *Journal of Child and Family Studies* 23 (2014): 548–557.
37 Darlow, Veronica, Jill M. Norvilitis, and Pamela Schuetze. "The relationship between helicopter parenting and adjustment to college." *Journal of Child and Family Studies* 26.8 (2017): 2291–2298.
38 Vinson, Kathleen. "Hovering too close: The ramifications of helicopter parenting in higher education." *Georgia State University Law Review* 29 (2012): 423.
39 Panova, Tayana, and Xavier Carbonell. "Is smartphone addiction really an addiction?" *Journal of Behavioral Addictions* 7.2 (2018): 252–259.
40 Palm, Fredrik. "Lacanian psychoanalysis, addiction and enjoyment." *Body & Society* 29.1 (2023): 56–78.
41 Freud, Sigmund. "Formulations regarding the two principles in mental functioning." *Organization and Pathology of Thought: Selected Sources.* Columbia University Press, 1951, 315–328.

42 Freud, Sigmund. *Three Essays on the Theory of Sexuality: The 1905 Edition*. Verso Books, 2017.
43 Potter-Efron, Ronald T., and Donald E. Efron. "Three models of shame and their relation to the addictive process." *Alcoholism Treatment Quarterly* 10.1–2 (1993): 23–48.
44 Lindstrom, Martin. "You love your iPhone. Literally." *New York Times* 1 (2011): 21A.
45 Dennis, Cindy-Lee, et al. "Screen use and internet addiction among parents of young children: A nationwide Canadian cross-sectional survey." *PLoS ONE* 17.1 (2022): e0257831.
46 Goh, Wendy W. L., Susanna Bay, and Vivian Hsueh-Hua Chen. "Young school children's use of digital devices and parental rules." *Telematics and Informatics* 32.4 (2015): 787–795.
47 Diefenbach, Sarah, and Kim Borrmann. "The smartphone as a pacifier and its consequences: Young adults' smartphone usage in moments of solitude and correlations to self-reflection." *Proceedings of the 2019 CHI Conference on Human Factors in Computing Systems*. New York: The Association for Computing Machinery, 2019.
48 Ahad, Annie Dayani, and Muhammad Anshari. "Smartphone habits among youth: Uses and gratification theory." *International Journal of Cyber Behavior, Psychology and Learning (IJCBPL)* 7.1 (2017): 65–75.
49 Muñoz, Cristóbal Fernández, Isidoro Arroyo Almaraz, and Francisco Garrcía García. "The effects of spontaneous use of smartphone on the attention and emotions of millennials students in a classroom." *International Linguistics Research* 2.2 (2019): p42–p42.
50 Alkis, Yunus, Zafer Kadirhan, and Mustafa Sat. "Development and validation of social anxiety scale for social media users." *Computers in Human Behavior* 72 (2017): 296–303.
51 Im, In-Chul, and Kyeung Jang. "The convergence influence of excessive smartphone use on attention deficit, learning environment, and academic procrastination in health college students." *Journal of the Korea Convergence Society* 8.12 (2017): 129–137.
52 Rohde, Luis Augusto, et al. "Attention-deficit/hyperactivity disorder in a diverse culture: Do research and clinical findings support the notion of a cultural construct for the disorder?" *Biological Psychiatry* 57.11 (2005): 1436–1441.
53 Samuels, Robert. *Generation X and the Rise of the Entertainment Subject*. Rowman & Littlefield, 2021.
54 Sutcliffe, Alistair G., Jens F. Binder, and Robin I. M. Dunbar. "Activity in social media and intimacy in social relationships." *Computers in Human Behavior* 85 (2018): 227–235.
55 Samuels, Robert, and Robert Samuels. "The pleasure principle and the death drive." *Freud for the Twenty-First Century: The Science of Everyday Life*. Springer, 2019, 17–25.
56 Maris, Cees. "Pornography is going on-line: The harm principle in Dutch law." *Law, Democracy & Development* 17.1 (2013): 1–23.
57 Arabatzis, Georgios. "Pornography and stress." *Conatus-Journal of Philosophy* 7.2 (2022): 143–156.
58 Wright, Paul J., et al. "Pornography and sexual dissatisfaction: The role of pornographic arousal, upward pornographic comparisons, and preference for pornographic masturbation." *Human Communication Research* 47.2 (2021): 192–214.
59 Snoek, Anke, et al. "Managing shame and guilt in addiction: A pathway to recovery." *Addictive Behaviors* 120 (2021): 106954.
60 Lewis, Marc. *The Biology of Desire: Why Addiction Is Not a Disease*. PublicAffairs, 2015.
61 LaBrie, Joseph W., et al. "Sexual experience and risky alcohol consumption among incoming first-year college females." *Journal of Child & Adolescent Substance Abuse* 20.1 (2010): 15–33.
62 Carlson, Scott R., Season C. Johnson, and Pauline C. Jacobs. "Disinhibited characteristics and binge drinking among university student drinkers." *Addictive Behaviors* 35.3 (2010): 242–251.

63 Buffardi, Laura E., and W. Keith Campbell. "Narcissism and social networking web sites." *Personality and Social Psychology Bulletin* 34.10 (2008): 1303–1314.

64 Samuels, Robert. "Neuroscience and the repression of psychoanalysis." *(Mis) Understanding Freud with Lacan, Zizek, and Neuroscience*. Cham: Springer International Publishing, 2022, 29–62.

65 Kim, Deokju. "Cognitive behavioral therapy for college students with smartphone addiction." *International Journal of Advanced Culture Technology* 9.4 (2021): 29–39.

66 Twenge, Jean M., and W. Keith Campbell. *The Narcissism Epidemic: Living in the Age of Entitlement*. Simon and Schuster, 2009.

67 Miller, Joshua D., et al. "Narcissism today: What we know and what we need to learn." *Current Directions in Psychological Science* 30.6 (2021): 519–525.

68 Kienast, Thorsten, et al. "Borderline personality disorder and comorbid addiction: Epidemiology and treatment." *Deutsches Ärzteblatt International* 111.16 (2014): 280.

69 King, Brian. *The Borderline Personality and the Culture of Materialism*. Alliant International University, San Francisco Bay, 2010.

70 Scott, Graham G., et al. "Posting photos on Facebook: The impact of narcissism, social anxiety, loneliness, and shyness." *Personality and Individual Differences* 133 (2018): 67–72.

71 Barry, Christopher T., et al. " 'Let me take a selfie': Associations between self-photography, narcissism, and self-esteem." *Psychology of Popular Media Culture* 6.1 (2017): 48.

72 Burgess, J. Peter, et al. "For want of not: Lacan's conception of anxiety." *Politics of Anxiety* (2017): 17–36.

73 Oleson, Kathryn C., et al. "Subjective overachievement: Individual differences in self-doubt and concern with performance." *Journal of Personality* 68.3 (2000): 491–524.

74 Gelfman, Morris. "Narcissism." *American Journal of Psychotherapy* 22.2 (1968): 296–303.

75 Kline, Paul. "Obsessional traits, obsessional symptoms and anal erotism." *The Experimental Study of Freudian Theories (Psychology Revivals)*. Routledge, 2013, 86–101.

76 Lacan, Jacques. *Family Complexes in the Formation of the Individual*. Antony Rowe, 2002.

77 Lacan, Jacques, Alan Sheridan, and Malcolm Bowie. "Aggressivity in psychoanalysis." *Écrits: A Selection*. Routledge, 2020, 9–32.

78 Dolezal, Luna. "Body shame and female experience." *The Body and Shame. Phenomenology, Feinism and the Socially Shaped Body*. Transcript Press, 2015, 103–122.

79 Block, Jennifer A. *Acceptance or* Change of Private Experiences: A Comparative Analysis in College Students with Public Speaking Anxiety*. State University of New York at Albany, 2002.

80 Freud, Sigmund. *Beyond the Pleasure Principle*. Penguin UK, 2003.

81 Read, Jennifer P., et al. "Rates of DSM–IV–TR trauma exposure and posttraumatic stress disorder among newly matriculated college students." *Psychological Trauma: Theory, Research, Practice, and Policy* 3.2 (2011): 148.

82 Sleep, Chelsea E., et al. "Narcissism and response validity: Do individuals with narcissistic features underreport psychopathology?" *Psychological Assessment* 29.8 (2017): 1059.

83 Joseph, Rhawn. "Awareness, the origin of thought, and the role of conscious self-deception in resistance and repression." *Psychological Reports* 46.3 (1980): 767–781.

84 de Groot, J. Lampl. "Inhibition and narcissism." *The Psychoanalytic Review (1913–1957)* 26 (1939): 114.

85 Hull, Mariam, and Mered Parnes. "Tics and TikTok: Functional tics spread through social media." *Movement Disorders Clinical Practice* 8.8 (2021): 1248–1252.

86 Giedinghagen, Andrea. "The tic in TikTok and (where) all systems go: Mass social media induced illness and Munchausen's by internet as explanatory models for social media associated abnormal illness behavior." *Clinical Child Psychology and Psychiatry* 28.1 (2023): 270–278.

87 Nagy, Péter, et al. "TikTok and tics: The possible role of social media in the exacerbation of tics during the COVID lockdown." *Ideggyogyaszati Szemle/Clinical Neuroscience* 75.5–6 (2022): 211–216.

88 Chodoff, Paul. "The diagnosis of hysteria: An overview." *American Journal of Psychiatry* 131.10 (1974): 1073–1078.

89 Stiglic, Gregor, Ruth Masterson Creber, and Leona Cilar Budler. "Internet use and psychosomatic symptoms among university students: Cross-sectional study." *International Journal of Environmental Research and Public Health* 19.3 (2022): 1774.

90 Grant, Alexandra F., et al. "Detecting feigned symptoms of depression, anxiety, and ADHD, in college students with the structured inventory of malingered symptomatology." *Applied Neuropsychology: Adult* 29.4 (2022): 443–451.

91 Khan, Sarah, Mona El Kouatly Kambris, and Hamda Alfalahi. "Perspectives of university students and faculty on remote education experiences during COVID-19-a qualitative study." *Education and Information Technologies* 27.3 (2022): 4141–4169.

Chapter 3

The Past and Present of Trauma-Informed Teaching

This chapter looks at the history and current use of what is now called trauma-informed pedagogy in order to articulate the main motivations and effects of this educational strategy.[1] Although my focus is on the field of college writing, much of the discussion can be applied to many other disciplines and aspects of contemporary society. The main argument is that a misguided understanding of trauma and therapy threatens to undermine higher education in particular and modern society in general. Through a careful reading of Michelle Day's dissertation "Wounds and Writing: Building Trauma-Informed Approaches to Writing Pedagogy," I expose the roots of a destructive educational ideology.[2]

Expanding Trauma

Day begins her text by focusing on how her work is driven by an awareness of how much students are suffering today:

> Since I began teaching in 2013, I've been surprised about how much personal distress my students have managed while taking my class. Parents have died before or during college after long battles with cancer. Friends have been killed in drunk driving accidents. Long-term romantic partnerships have ended dramatically, disrupting living arrangements and social support systems. Students have become temporarily homeless, gone to rehab while still trying to finish the semester, or contracted serious illnesses or injuries. They've been sexually assaulted or abused by a loved one. They've struggled through long custody battles with former partners and tried to write papers while their children were in the hospital. They've had PTSD from wartime duties; they've struggled with anxiety and depression, sometimes to the point of suicidal thoughts. As I worked with these students, it became clear how trauma and distress are common and central components of students' college experiences. These difficult stories also increased my felt sense that being generally empathetic toward students and their trauma was not good enough, if I wanted to be an effective teacher; as educators, we must teach the real people actually in front of us, and the more we understand about today's

DOI: 10.4324/9781003545668-3

college students, the more we understand how trauma impacts their educational well-being.

(1)

The first thing that we have to ask in relation to this representation of contemporary students is if students today are suffering more from trauma than past cohorts. After all, we know that people have never lived longer, more protected lives than now.[3] We also know that rates of crime and violent death have been massively decreased over previous centuries, and many past forms of abuse and exploitation have been outlawed.[4] While traumatic events still occur in people's lives, it would be hard to argue that things have gotten worse on average for most people. The question we are then forced to ask is if trauma is being noticed more than before or if its rate of incidence is being exaggerated.[5]

It is, of course, difficult to challenge another person's suffering, but it is important to realize that if we want to claim that most students have been traumatized, we have to ask how trauma is actually being defined.[6] We also have to question whether the goal of education is to be therapeutic. Clearly, Day believes that most of her students – if not all of them – have been victims of trauma and that her role as a teacher is to provide empathy in relation to student suffering.[7] If we think that the rate of trauma is being exaggerated and the role of teachers is being misdirected, then we should ask how we get to this point. My most basic response is that a combination of not understanding the goals of modern education coupled with the repression of psychoanalysis has enabled a counter-productive model of therapy to replace effective education.

As Day points out, she is not the only one who thinks that most college students today are victims of trauma: "Several recent studies at major U.S. universities indicate that at least half and as many as 85% of college students have experienced one or more traumatic events (Vrana et al; Pritchard et al; Moser et al; Carello and Butler" (2). Like all surveys, the first issue is how trauma is being defined and how reliable the collected data is. Since these polls rely on self-reporting, we run into the problem of how the students are themselves understanding the meaning of trauma and whether they are being accurate in their responses to survey questions.[8]

The Psychoanalytic Understanding of Hysteria, Trauma, and Narcissism

From a psychoanalytic perspective, every person has been traumatized by the social imposition of morality.[9] In fact, Freud first thought that all of his hysterical patients were sexually assaulted by their fathers, and then he came to believe that some of them only imagined that they were abused.[10] However, his final position was that trauma is a universal experience caused by the imposition of social morality in relation to our sexual and violent impulses.[11] Yet, he also focused on how people responded to trauma, and these responses shaped their basic relationship with others and themselves. What most people, then, misunderstand about trauma is its relationship to hysteria, and what defines hysteria is how suffering is used in order to gain an identity and influence others in an indirect, unconscious way.[12] I have called this relation between identity and others the "victim complex" in order to stress how the expression of suffering to others allows one to see oneself as innocent and good, as others are represented as being evil perpetrators.[13] This development of a polarized perspective enables the victim to feel that any revenge is justified and all criticism should be disallowed.[14]

Of course, the theory of the victim complex can look like it is simply blaming the victim, but what psychoanalysis offers is a method to examine why and how people might use their victim status to manipulate others on an unconscious emotional level. In fact, an analysis of Freud's case of Dora reveals that he derived his concept of "secondary gain" to account for the ways the suffering subject uses their complaints to gain emotional leverage over others.[15] After all, it is hard to criticize someone who is suffering, and real and imagined pain can be used as an excuse to avoid undesired social obligations. Moreover, by taking on the status of being a victim, one gives oneself a stable identity and an explanation for one's own life.[16] Freud also found that people often learn how to be victims by copying others, and in this form of empathy, identification occurs on an unconscious level.[17] From this perspective, empathy cannot be the cure for trauma and suffering since empathy is itself a form of hysterical identification.[18]

The origins of Freud's theory of hysteria can be traced back to his early *Project for a Scientific Psychology* where he examines how when a baby cries and the parent responds with help, the child learns that the expression of suffering is the way to get others to supply recognition, love, and knowledge.[19] Thus, the underlying desire is to have the self recognized and cared for, and this requires the other to understand what the signs of suffering mean.[20] On a fundamental level, when people come to therapy or analysis, what they really want is to have their suffering verified by the other, but what Freud quickly learned is that this demand to be saved by others creates a relationship of dependency, which he later labeled as transference.[21] Importantly, Freud also learned that transference is both the biggest enabler and obstacle to analysis. Since people want to be saved by an idealized caregiver, they become dependent on an all-powerful person who makes them even more insecure and dependent. The trick of psychoanalytic treatment concerns how the analyst both enables and moves beyond the transference.

In contrast to psychoanalysis, most forms of therapy do nothing to remove the transference; in fact, they often enhance it as the therapist is placed in the position of the one who knows and cares.[22] One reason for this feeding of dependency is that the therapist enjoys being idealized, and also, this relationship feeds the narcissism of the therapist. As Lacan was fond of pointing out, the narcissist seeks to have the ideal ego verified by others, and one way this is achieved in therapy is by believing that one's empathy proves that one is a good person.[23] Like the parent who seeks to make all of the child's suffering and problems go away, the therapist, as a good maternal figure, seeks to be recognized for being knowing and caring.[24] On the most basic level, the hysteric desires to be recognized for suffering, while the narcissist seeks to have the ideal self verified. It is important to stress here that what Freud called obsessional neurosis is usually now diagnosed as a narcissistic personality disorder.[25]

What we are seeing in parenting, education, and society as a whole is that social institutions are taking on the role of the narcissistic caregiver who recognizes the suffering of hysterical subjects. In other words, there has never been a greater need for psychoanalysis, but psychoanalytic theory and treatment are being undermined by misguided notions of biological determinism, Cognitive Behavioral Therapy, and other forms of non-analytic therapy.[26] In terms of higher education, some teachers and administrators want to see themselves as being good, virtuous people, and so they cater to the hysteria of their students, and the result is not only an undermining of education but also an attack on reason itself.

Misreading Freud

Returning to Day's text, we discover how a misunderstanding of psychoanalysis has led to a promotion of trauma as a key to higher education: "Freud and Janet, working at the same time, were among the first to posit female hysteria as 'a condition caused by psychological trauma. Unbearable emotional reactions to traumatic events produced an altered state of consciousness, which in turn induced the hysteria symptoms' (Herman 12). Trauma at this time meant 'the wounding of the mind brought about by sudden, unexpected, emotional shock' that shatters the personality, as epitomized by the hysterical female" (6). What is missed in this discussion of Freud's early theory of hysteria and trauma is the fact that he eventually distinguished between neurosis based on trauma and the hysterical secondary gain from suffering. In the case of what he called "war neurosis," traumatic shocks result in flashbacks and other forms of unsymbolized repetition, while in the case of hysteria, the emphasis is on how suffering is used on an unconscious level to establish a sense of identity and to influence others.[27] By equating hysteria and trauma, the difference between the uncontrolled repetition of an unexpected event and the retroactive rewriting of suffering is lost. In other words, there is a great deal of difference between what we now call PTSD and Freud's conception of hysteria.

Day continues this misunderstanding of psychoanalysis by focusing on Freud's earliest model of therapy: "Hysteria's power, they suggested, stemmed from repression of painful memories, and treatment thus involved "recovering" those memories from the subconscious in an altered state guided by a therapist ("hypnosis"). In other words, Freud found that "hysterics suffered mainly from reminiscences" and healed only after putting those reminiscences into words" (6). The problem with this representation of psychoanalysis is that it fails to mention how Freud gave up his cathartic method because he realized that it often had no lasting effects, and one reason why it did not help in the long run is that it fed – instead of removing – the transference.[28] By acting as the one who knows how to fix the problem, the analyst ends up being idealized, and this idealization not only increases dependency but also blocks the overcoming of repression.[29] While it is true that Freud thought that hysterics suffered from their memories, he also thought that these memories were distorted by substitution and displacement. It is, therefore, fantasy that produces symptoms, but fantasy is itself a defense against reality.[30]

Although Day does touch on the relations among hysteria, trauma, fantasy, and memory, she does not understand the concept of secondary gain: "Earlier in his studies, Freud suggested that sexual exploitation was at the core of hysteria, but he later argued that such hysteria was related in large part to repressed infantile wishes and fantasies (the basis of much psychoanalytic theory), which modern feminist theorists like Herman have rejected as denying the significance of actual trauma on the individual psyche, though others found much explanatory power in psychoanalytic concepts, such as projection" (6). Since many feminist critics and analysts reject the idea that women might imagine their trauma, they prevent us from seeing how suffering can be used as an unconscious mode of identity and social interaction.[31]

Unintentionally, Day does point to the problem of equating war neurosis with hysteria when she discusses how our understanding of trauma has developed:

Though support for researching trauma has waxed and waned over the years, two historical moments in the 1900s solidified its validity as an area of inquiry and have shaped modern uses of the term: World War I and the era after the Vietnam War. During and after World War I, many soldiers experienced "shell shock," or combat-related neuroses that appeared similar to the symptoms of "hysterical women." Though some still accused shell-shocked soldiers of malingering or otherwise having defective moral character (including being "weak like women"), medical professionals re-ignited interest in discovering how even the best soldiers might be overcome by the terror of war and how recovering repressed memories, among other treatments, might bring catharsis and allow them to return to military duty (Herman 21).

(7)

As the passage reveals, our comprehension of trauma has been, in part, blocked by the false equivalence drawn between hysteria and war neurosis (PTSD).[32] With hysteria, suffering is expressed in order to gain a sense of identity and to influence others on an unconscious level, while with war neurosis, the central problem is that the shocking event has not been integrated into the unconscious mind. Since, as Lacan states, the Real of trauma is impossible to symbolize, memories return in the form of an unsymbolized image in external reality.[33]

As we shall see throughout this book, a major issue shaping how trauma is understood and dealt with on college campuses concerns the way different diagnostic categories are defined.[34] This lack of clear definition is apparent in the way that PTSD has been described:

Efforts by activist groups to demonstrate how trauma is an epidemic – rather than the narrow experience of a few weaker minded groups of people – contributed to a turning point in trauma's history: the *Diagnostic and Statistical Manual-III* (begun in 1974 and published in 1980) included Post-Traumatic Stress Disorder for the first time. This meant that PTSD, and therefore trauma, became a more publicly-ratified, diagnosable condition with identifiable symptoms, impacts, and treatment options across the types of terror (e.g. war, rape, abuse, disaster) that might cause this condition.

(7)

In calling trauma an epidemic, Day points to the fact that a non-psychoanalytic definition has enabled the concept to spread without control as it infects other forms of mental disorder.[35] Since any extreme event can be considered to be traumatic, and the unconscious responses of individuals to these events are not considered, the definition of PTSD becomes shaped by personal, political, and cultural concerns.[36]

One of the effects of these expansive definitions of trauma and PTSD in higher education is that they enable a wide range of disciplines to take up this topic: "Once trauma received validation in this way, more disciplines began to import the concept in their own fields, especially in humanities disciplines, where attention to issues of representation, narrative, and memory are central. In part, this turn was predictable, since Freud had long argued that trauma's force made it nearly incommunicable, and his work involved finding ways to help patients recover the painful memories and put them into words" (7). Of course, one of the main problems with this importation of trauma into different disciplines was that every teacher was now called on to act as a therapist – even the ones lacking any therapeutic training or experience.[37]

Healing Trauma

A paradox of employing trauma in diverse disciplines is that many of the advocates for this move are attracted to the notion that trauma represents a failure of representation: "Theorists in trauma studies often describe trauma in apocalyptic language and focus on the problems it creates for memory and representation (Berger). For example, Cathy Caruth – [explains] that trauma is 'the response to an unexpected or overwhelming violent event or events that are not fully grasped as they occur, but return later in repeated flashbacks, nightmares, and other repetitive phenomena'" (8). In stressing the repeated failure to symbolize traumatic events, these humanities scholars appear to revel in the failures of language and other forms of symbolization, which is ironic since their main occupation is to understand symbolic representations.[38] Perhaps this self-consuming ideology points to a narcissistic need to conform to social norms and forms while one leaves a space for individual differences and authenticity. Another possibility is that a focus on trauma provides a perverse enjoyment of the perceived suffering of others.[39]

In the teaching of college writing, trauma has played an important role in many different areas:

Writing studies scholars have engaged trauma in an impressively diverse range of composition pedagogy and rhetorical scholarship. Key threads in this history include efforts: to see students confront difficult and important social issues, like xenophobia or genocide (Ames; Marbach; Payne); to help students use writing to heal from distressing or traumatic circumstances (Harris; Bishop; MacCurdy; Bracher "Writing Cure"); to combat the silence that often accompanies trauma (Cole; Kaufman; Thompson); to discuss and promote ethical representation and reception of others' trauma (Hesford); to help promote transformative learning through educational "crisis" moments (Bracher; Britzman and Pitt); and other purposes.

(12–13)

This focus on cultural and individual trauma represents a strong impulse of educators to see their students as suffering, which, in turn, places the teacher in the position of one who is supposed to help heal personal and social problems.[40] It is my argument that this expansive definition of trauma and therapy crowds out the core mission of college composition courses to teach students how to communicate in a more effective manner.[41] Moreover, by privileging emotion over reason, the entire foundation of modern science and education is called into question.

Instead of teachers seeing their role as helping students to learn, they are now often representing themselves as healers: "Regardless of purpose, this literature – especially work focused on pedagogy – frequently argues for the healing potential of writing for individuals and society in ways that function on an anemic understanding of trauma, as well as overemphasizing the place of a single writing classroom in promoting healing, which neglects ecological perspectives on trauma/ resilience and practical considerations for ethically interacting with survivors" (13). In representing students as survivors and teachers as promoting healing, a new vision of education is presented. Furthermore, while the term "survivor" once represented individuals who were traumatic victims of the Holocaust, now the term is being applied to almost every student.[42]

One of the more questionable practices that has resulted from the expansive definitions of trauma, survivor, and therapy concerns the effort to get students to write about their most upsetting personal experiences: "Jeffrey Berman advocates for 'risky writing,' or opportunities for students to write about trauma – from rape to encountering racial prejudice to loss of a loved one – asking them to self-disclose stories that are typically shrouded in secrecy and shame. He proposes a few strategies to minimize risk of these disclosures – such as teaching the importance of empathy – so that students can work through such difficult experiences through writing (e.g. the 'writing cure)" (14).[43] A notion guiding this form of personal composition is the idea that people can be healed by simply writing about a difficult event.[44] By motivating students to represent their traumas for an empathic teacher, not only are students subjected to people with little training as therapists, but it becomes hard for an instructor to assess the work of someone who is presenting their suffering.

Some teachers who embrace trauma-based pedagogy have also used their positions to take on social issues from a progressive or Left-leaning perspective: "A more recent turn within this "writing-as-healing-for-society" paradigm comes from service-learning or community engagement scholarship, which has suggested that

writing about trauma in the context of community work can promote societal healing through greater critical understanding of others' trauma and building empathy
across difference" (16). Once again, an important issue to examine is: why are
these teachers not focusing on teaching writing?[45] There is also the problem of turning the classroom into a space for political indoctrination. From a psychoanalytic
perspective, we can understand this movement through the idea that obsessional
narcissists want to prove to themselves that they are good people, and the way that
they do this is by having their good acts and intentions recognized by others. In
representing themselves as healers, these pseudo-therapists and social activists take
on the idealized role of being the good mother for their suffering students as they
act to bring comfort to a sick society that needs to be healed.[46]

For Day, the problem is not that these teachers are acting as if they are therapists, the problem is that their understanding of trauma and healing is derived from
psychoanalysis and not clinical social work: "These insufficiencies stem from the
way writing studies has tended to draw much more heavily on the psychoanalytical
and trauma studies concepts that have some explanatory power for our work with
students but ignoring the clinical literature that examines exactly how, under what
circumstances, and with what ethical practices these pedagogies might be experienced as healing rather than ineffective or, at worst, harmful" (17). As an example
of the repression of psychoanalysis, this turn to clinical social work plays the dual
role of debasing Freud and idealizing a mode of social intervention that relies on a
pre-psychoanalytic comprehension of psychopathology and treatment.[47]

One of the reasons why Day and others may be turning to ineffective theories
and models of therapy and social intervention is that they want to be able to say that
they are not only healing individuals, but they are also healing society:

> Furthermore, the field's explorations on trauma so far often neglect an ecological
> perspective on trauma and resilience, even when acknowledging the systemic
> inequalities that perpetuate trauma. According to Dass-Brailsford, ecological
> perspectives on trauma view violence as ecological threats that "threaten the
> capacity of communities to promote health," and they also "assume that mental
> health issues are influenced by multiple intersecting factors, which include indi-
> vidual characteristics, family, school, community, and other contexts."
>
> (18)

Of course, Freud also argued that a person's mental health is affected by family,
culture, and other social influences; however, since these critiques of psychoanalysis often have little understanding of this field, they simply see Freud as only focusing on the isolated individual.[48] While it should be clear that psychoanalysis is not a
form of education or politics, Freud's fundamental concepts help us to explain both
of these social institutions.[49]

As Day reveals, psychoanalysis is often repressed because the focus is now
on empathy as the key to individual and social healing: "Baumgartner and Dis-
cher and Pignetti contend that students can be taught to be ethical, critical social

actors working against trauma in the context of *a* service-learning course where they develop empathy" (18–19). Many scholars inside and outside of the humanities believe that the key to helping individuals and societies is to use empathy, but from a psychoanalytic perspective, empathy often only reinforces symptoms, repression, defense mechanisms, and self-destructive drives.[50] The point of analysis is to get people to discover new things about themselves through the process of free association and the working through of the transference: The goal is not to have the patient feel that the analyst is a good parent who loves and understands them. Unfortunately, many current modes of therapy and education have replaced analysis with empathy, and while this may help the healers feel like they are doing the right thing, there is little evidence that this type of relationship can get to the underlying causes of human suffering and aggression.[51]

As Day indicates, when teachers center their classes on getting students to confess their traumas, these instructors can end up doing great harm to the people they are trying to help: "Though the scholars referenced above explore the benefits of students disclosing trauma in the classroom (at times suggesting we should invite these disclosures), there remains much less (if any) discussion regarding research-validated principles and practices for instructors responding to these disclosures, nor has there been adequate rendering of possible risks to students" (19). By motivating untrained teachers to act as therapists, students are placed in a vulnerable position as the instructors can use their classroom authority to influence what students say and do. In fact, this combination of eliciting the reporting of traumas in a context where one person holds most of the power leads to cult-like group formations.[52] As Freud discovered, at the foundation of most extreme groups, we find individuals regressing to the position of a helpless infant in front of an idealized power.[53]

Even if these therapist-teachers avoid using their positions to manipulate students, there is still the problem of instructors burning out because of the multiple demands that are being placed on them:

> Additionally, there is very little discussion of day-to-day concerns such as warding against compassion fatigue, or mandatory reporting policies, which may require instructors to break confidentiality with their students and which may actually endanger students (for example, if it results in an investigation in which an abuser becomes aware that the victim has told their secret). There is also little attention to the role of triggering – how sensory reminders of a traumatic experience can cause an individual to re-experience the original trauma as if it were actually happening – and how to help students who are emotionally overwhelmed to calm down.
>
> (19–20)

While in some rare cases, students suffering from PTSD can be triggered by course material and lessons, for the most part, the larger issue is how teachers promote reason and equality in a situation where each student is seen as having their own pressing emotional needs.[54]

The Politics of Trauma-Informed Pedagogy

In having students write about their personal suffering, teachers may become unable to fairly judge their work:

> Finally, the uptake of this limited scholarship in teaching practice has privileged the "powerful," "moving," or "honest" personal narrative about trauma in ways that are misleading. Ann Ruggles Gere locates this trope in personal writing pedagogies of the 1980s, in which personal writing – thought to elicit a more authentic writerly voice – often resulted in students telling their instructors stories about traumatic experiences. These trauma narratives appeared in scholarship and collections that publish student work, and the literature suggests instructors also give accolades in class to the students who produce these narratives.
>
> (20)

This relation between the suffering student and the rewarding teacher replicates the dynamic between the hysterical complaint and the narcissistic response: Instructors want to feel good about themselves by caring for students who display their psychic pain.[55] As we see with student essays in college applications, the focus on being empathetic to expressed trauma can result in the lost ability to make fair and equal judgments.[56] Thus, one of the things that critics reject about Diversity, Equity, and Inclusion policies and practices is that they harm the effort to assess and credit ability and expertise.[57]

As Day points out, students are trained at an early age how to give teachers what they desire, and so an instructor who wants to see expressions of suffering will often feed the students' efforts to please the teacher in order to get a higher grade:

> One problem with this trend is that it claims to prove what it cannot – that students who write about their trauma and express some degree of healing through writing have actually healed from trauma, for good, when clinical literature suggests healing is an uneven and cyclical process, sometimes a journey that never quite reaches its destination. Furthermore, research on literacy narratives has indicated that students are quite savvy at knowing what narratives professors expect and performing accordingly (Williams; Webb-Sunderhaus). Thus, it is difficult to determine what benefits, if any, a student has received from discussions or written prompts that engage trauma and to what extent the student may be repeating the "powerful personal narrative" that the instructor wants to hear.
>
> (20–21)

In this type of hysterical transference, students display their traumas so that they can receive the praise and validation of an authority figure. As psychoanalysis has taught us, one of the risks of this dynamic is that teachers can abuse their power by taking advantage of their role in recognizing student helplessness.[58] Even though many of these teachers would like to believe that they are trying not to act as an authority, their ability to judge and grade students gives them a power they cannot simply ignore. Of course, one current strategy is simply to not grade or assess students, but this lack of judgment and criticism serves the purpose of placing the narcissistic instructor in the position of the Other, who simply reinforces the underlying transferential desire for love, recognition, and knowledge.[59]

While there has been a backlash against trauma-informed pedagogy outside and inside of higher education, the people rejecting this type of education are often doing it for purely political reasons:

> Faculty and university administration pushed back against calls for trigger warnings, arguing that they impede intellectual freedom (Bass and Clark; Bianco; Cooper), coddle students from the realities of adulthood (Halberstam; Essig), prevent real and substantial learning (Boostrom; Cooper; Essig), mark an attempt by students not to be challenged (Boostrom; Cooper; Essig; Bianco), and reflect neoliberal co-opting and individualizing of traumas at the expense of more structural causes.
>
> (22)

Day highlights here many of the real problems caused by trauma-informed pedagogy, yet she continues to endorse it. Here, we encounter a problem of ironic conformity – where people know that what they are doing is wrong, yet they continue to do it because they feel that their awareness of the problem prevents them from being responsible for it.[60] Therefore, Day may point out how this type of education harms students, teachers, and education itself, but she still insists that it is a vital form of instruction.

In one of her attempts to both accept and reject the criticism of trauma-informed pedagogy, Day seeks to rationalize the undermining of reason, science, merit, expertise, standards, and discipline: "Concerns about coddling students stem from justifiable concerns about academic rigor, intellectual freedom, and instructor autonomy; however, these concerns also conflate discomfort with triggering, misrepresent the nature of retraumatization and its impact on academic success, oversimplify the concept of classroom safety, and ultimately exclude the perspectives of traumatized students from the classroom space" (39). In this effort to justify a focus on students who have been traumatized, Day both reveals and conceals issues concerning academic standards and emotional manipulation. While teachers are not therapists or parents, they are often asked to play these roles by responding to student suffering instead of concentrating on producing and communicating scientific reason.[61]

Even in writing courses and other humanities disciplines, teachers should seek to apply the scientific method by privileging evidence, reason, and impartiality, but what we often find instead is an emphasis on personal experience and feelings.[62]

As Day points out, this focus on emotions places teachers in the position of being therapists who know that they are not therapists:

> "Teachers aren't therapists" became a touchstone in this conversation, as both an oppositional reaction by skeptics and an obligatory nod by proponents of pedagogies that attempted to leverage writing's healing potential. Several important realities inform the admonition that teachers are not, and should not try to be, therapists. These include: instructors should not tamper with psychological processes they don't understand; an over-focus on the personal can promote navel-gazing and individualism at the expense of academic (and) writing development; directly engaging students' trauma can create several ethical and liability issues; and so on. However, this chapter also demonstrates how this truism does not adequately reflect the nature of writing instructors' work with students, our role in students' mental health, our responsibilities for creating effective learning environments, and the skills instructors feel they need to work effectively and ethically with students who are in distress.
>
> (40)

Here, we find an example of what Freud called negation: Day presents many of the problems with trauma-informed pedagogy, but she clings to the idea that none of these affirmed issues really matter.[63] Since she believes that we need to teach students who are distressed in a different way, she cannot escape from the desire to place instructors in a therapeutic position.

One way that Day is able to justify this type of pedagogy is by pointing to an extreme reaction to extreme forms of sensitive teaching:

> Many administrators and instructors argued passionately against trigger warnings in particular, making trigger warnings perhaps the most high-profile example of broader discussions about psychological safety at college. Fears circulated about how trigger warnings – especially if *required* by institutions – could impede intellectual freedom (Bass and Clark; Bianco; Cooper), coddle students from the realities of adulthood (Halberstam; Essig; Lukianoff and Haidt), prevent real and substantial learning (Boostrom; Cooper; Essig), allow students to avoid being challenged (Boostrom; Cooper; Essig; Bianco), and reflect neoliberal co-opting and individualizing of traumas at the expense of more structural causes (Halberstam; Alvarez and Schneider; Cecire).
>
> (44)

While very few teachers probably use trigger warnings, the political Right has latched onto their employment because they represent a clear case of instructors limiting free speech by treating students in a protective manner.[64] Conservatives also fear the trigger warnings fail to expose students to harsh realities as they prevent students from being challenged in any way.[65]

The High Cost of Student Mental Health

As Day points out, one reason why there is a heightened concern for protecting the mental health of students is that an increasing number of them are coming to college with diagnosed mental disorders: "In part, conversations about psychological safety arose from the fact that more students than ever are able to attend college despite social, disability, or mental illness factors that historically have precluded them from postsecondary education (Pritchard; Carter; Price)" (45). We do not know if students are being over-diagnosed or if more of them are suffering from mental health issues, but what we do know is that institutions of higher education are spending a large amount of money on dealing with what they perceive to be a student mental health crisis.[66]

A possible reason why these institutions are so invested in a costly response to student mental health issues is that they want to be seen as being caring and empathic, yet as Day partially admits, this huge attention to accommodation can undermine the foundations of education itself:

> To some educators, student requests for trigger warnings, safe spaces, or other accommodations (such as alternate assignments, forgiving absence policies) only serve to further erode the purpose and goals of a college education, rather than helping traumatized students learn more effectively. Psychological safety, they argue, opposes education, which is inherently uncomfortable, challenging, and painful. In other words, students don't need to be coddled in "safe classrooms." Instead, they need to grow up.
>
> (45)

The way that the critics of the current problem are presented appears to be a rhetorical effort to make them sound simply heartless and mean. Yet, many of the faculty resisting this movement are not doing it because they are afraid of coddling sensitive students or because they simply do not care about student suffering – the real issue is that a focus on individual trauma makes it hard to teach all of the students in a fair and equal manner.

When teachers cater to individual students, they often create a situation where different standards are applied according to the instructor's personal feelings and attitudes. For example, Day refers to a teacher who started to question the preferential treatment of particular students: "James described one student who was dealing with a variety of past and current trauma and how James both desired to help this student succeed and feared that he was 'winding up creating an individual set of rules for this one student'" (46). Thus, in the effort to help a particular student, what can be lost is any sense of a universal standard and the equal treatment of each person.[67] Day also relates that some instructors she interviewed felt that the emphasis on trauma could create a situation where students are harmed: "Another instructor – Thor – questions whether making accommodations for traumatized students sometimes actually reinforces feelings of helplessness and dependency that trauma causes" (46). Since teachers never know how a particular student might react to encountering upsetting class material, instructors who believe that they comprehend a student's psychology may end up doing more harm than good.[68] It is also very difficult for a teacher to anticipate every student's individual mental health needs. Although Day points to some ways of trying to protect students, many of the recommended approaches undermine the basic foundations of effective instruction: "Jeffrey Berman, for example, describes elements of safety he uses to minimize the risks of personal writing in his 'risky writing classrooms,' such as empathy, grading pass/fail, allowing anonymity, weekly conferences, and so on" (47). This idea of grading students on a pass/fail basis points to one of the ways that a focus on trauma and emotion can harm educational standards and assessment.[69]

As Day indicates, some faculty feel that education should not be centered on safety since students have to encounter new and possibly upsetting knowledge: "Liam Corley discusses classroom strategies aimed at welcoming, relevant, and excellent instruction that consists of discussions that are rarely 'safe, comfortable, or predictable' so that students do not stagnate in safeness" (48). If modern education is about learning new things that transcend what people already know, then the focus on protecting students can undermine instruction from within.

Diversity and Trauma

The roots of this current emphasis on trauma-informed pedagogy can be tracked back in part to the diversifying of higher education admissions: "In fact, the tradition of understanding and valuing "different" student experiences can be traced back to the field's scholarship in the 1970s and 1980s, when open admissions policies meant a diversifying student body that necessitated new pedagogical theories and practices to account for who it was exactly that instructors were teaching and how those identities meant they know/learn differently" (49). With the advent of open admissions, universities and colleges had to learn how to enroll and satisfy a diverse group of students with a wide range of skills and knowledge.[70] One of the responses to this diversity was the now-common notion that students learn best from people who share the same social identity.[71] However, by catering to specific racial and ethnic groups, these schools harmed the universality of science and the equality of modern democracy. In other words, the notion that students and teachers were defined by their particular identities meant that there could be no universal, impersonal subject, and this lack of universality makes it hard to treat everyone equally or to approach material from an unbiased perspective.[72]

Instead of trying to make education accessible to everyone by giving them the same tools and opportunities, the goal of many Equity, Diversity, and Inclusion programs is to treat each group differently.[73] One reason for this unequal treatment is the idea that since students come from unequal educational and familial backgrounds, efforts should be made to give the disadvantaged special accommodations.[74] While this type of policy makes administrators and faculty feel good about helping these students, it undermines the foundations of modern science and democracy by replacing the universal subject with a particular group or individual. Complicating matters is the notion that different groups have also suffered distinct traumas, and so in order to help these minoritized people, it is necessary to focus on emotion, personal experience, and trauma: "Trauma represents a salient and prevalent factor of difference/identity that deserves more explicit attention in literature on inclusive writing pedagogies, as does psychological safety, as a possible pedagogical response designed to be inclusive of that difference" (49). Since many minority-based social movements on the Left produce empathy and solidarity by rallying around a shared trauma, there is an overlap between faculty seeking to use their classroom for progressive political reasons and ones representing themselves as therapists dealing with student mental health issues.[75]

While many on the Right have attacked higher education for trying to indoctrinate students into a Left-wing ideology, the bigger problem is that the focus on both group and individual trauma can create a learning environment that prevents actual learning: "Participants were weary of how forgiving absences/late work or providing students alternative assignments might undermine the rigor of their courses, and though they all valued listening when students discussed personal distress, they also questioned whether this could distract from accomplishing course goals and take too much of their own emotional energy" (53). By asking our teachers to be political activists and therapists, we are often crowding out the attention that should be paid to teaching students how to apply reason through shared methods and empirical testing. Moreover, one effect has been grade inflation and the reluctance of teachers to upset students by giving them accurate feedback on their work.[76]

As a university instructor, I can attest to the difficulty of trying to accommodate particular students while maintaining shared, transparent, and fair standards: "Most participants also stated that instructors' primary responsibility is to educate, not counsel, and thus it's necessary to set limits on some accommodations, including trigger warnings, in order to protect the integrity of the educational space and avoid encouraging students to "stay stuck" in their trauma" (53–54). This balancing of accommodation and educational rigor is easier said than done, and many educators resolve this conflict by simply giving every student high praise and high grades.[77] In fact, the use of student evaluations to assess teachers motivates many faculty members to do anything they can to accommodate their students, and with the rising number of non-tenure-track faculty, this problem is only increased since these teachers are often assessed only by student evaluations.[78]

As Day points out, even when teachers do decide to cater to individual students because of their perceived suffering, the instructors may be doing more harm than good: "These feelings are somewhat supported by social work scholar Betty J. Barrett and sociologist Jack Mezirow, who have both argued that pedagogies that emphasize supporting students without sufficiently challenging them create dependent students who don't learn effectively learn, rather than psychologically safe ones" (54). If learning requires getting out of one's comfort zone, then teaching based on safety undermines the educational process itself.[79] Day adds that the faculty with the least amount of job security will suffer the most when they attempt to protect students through the use of trigger warnings and other defensive techniques: "In fact, both Bianco and the AAUP worry that administrative policies requiring trigger warnings would unfairly affect instructors with the least job security – adjuncts and other non-tenure-track instructors – by allowing students to file complaints that effectively censor instructors' course materials under penalty of being fired or receiving reduced course loads" (54–55). If students think that it is the role of teachers to not challenge them or have them encounter material they would prefer to avoid, then they may lash out at faculty without job security or academic freedom who fail to create what is considered to be a safe learning environment.[80]

Although trigger warnings have received a lot of public and political attention, these devices are only a small part of the general ideology concerning the imagined relation between traumatized students and accommodating instructors: "Jenny Jarvie writes that trigger warnings 'risk opening the door to a never-ending litany of requests,' even frivolous ones, such as a petition by Wellesley College students against a sculpture of a man in his underwear" (55). Students are not only complaining about what material they are exposed to in class, but they are also using their real and imagined suffering to ask to be excused from class attendance, participation, and testing.[81] Making matters worse is that during the COVID pandemic, many schools asked teachers to accept any and all requests for accommodation, and once the pandemic subsided, this lax institutional attitude was sometimes maintained.[82]

Although faculty and critics who question student excuses and complaints are often seen as being insensitive and mean, it is vital to realize that a key aspect of hysteria and the victim complex is that the person who expresses their suffering should not be critiqued, and if they are questioned, their aggression towards the critic will feel justified. After all, how can you attack a person who is lying in a hospital bed with cancer?[83] Of course, the book you are currently reading will be easily dismissed and criticized by people who are invested in trauma-informed pedagogy, but we need to look at valid research concerning the effectiveness of this type of education.[84] We also have to consider the experience of many faculty who are caught between the desire to uphold standards and the wish to help suffering students. As Day documents, a major issue concerns the ability to fairly grade students if they have made an emotional connection with their suffering: "For instance, Dr. Von discussed the need for boundaries with regard to hearing students' trauma stories, because, although compassion and listening are important, 'You don't wanna be emotionally blackmailed. You don't ever wanna be put in a position in which that emotion affects the grade you give'" (55). It simply is not fair to grade students differently based on how an individual teacher feels about an individual student.

Catering to students who are suffering or have mental issues can also make the job of teaching feel overwhelming and unworkable:

Cathy, who has been teaching more than 30 years, acknowledged a similar tension where some students become "excessively needy" and can take up too much of the instructors' time – something she had to learn to navigate as a younger teacher when a distressed student attended her office hours so often just to chat, that she was unable to give full attention to other aspects of her teaching. A long-time literature faculty member, James, worried about whether having so many accommodations for one particularly distressed student has created unfair practices that are not ultimately serving the students' education.

(55)

Although we may want to make sure that every student succeeds, it is unrealistic to think that untrained teachers can heal students during office hours or private sessions.[85] On a fundamental level, this dynamic between the empathic teacher and the traumatized student can undermine both the learning of the student and the mental health of the teacher.

A social side-effect of concentrating on perceived trauma and selective empathy is that the ability of different individuals and groups to work together or form political coalitions may be undermined in a competition between who suffers the most: "Educators also cite more subtle ways that trigger warnings might reinforce rather than combat injustices. For instance, Halberstam argues that trigger warnings usher in 'the re-emergence of a rhetoric of harm and trauma [could cast] all social difference in terms of hurt feelings and [divide] up politically allied subjects into hierarchies of roundedness'" (57). In fact, one of the problems facing the Democratic Party is that there are so many different groups seeking attention and special treatment that they have a hard time finding common ground.[86]

Trauma vs. Anxiety

A driving force behind the changing nature of education, therapy, and parenting is the growing power of women in all aspects of society. My argument here is not to criticize this important social revolution, but I do want to discuss how the privileging of maternal care over paternal authority has important ramifications.[87] In the case of trauma-informed pedagogy, some of the push to pay attention to student mental health and expressed suffering comes from females who connect the women's movement to an increased awareness of sexual assault and gender discrimination: "Essig argues that trigger warnings are directed toward protecting *women*, especially female survivors of sexual assault" (57). As Day indicates, due to the high level of reported sexual assault on college campuses, there has been an effort to prevent female students from being triggered by encountering rape-related material.[88] While this response to a horrible personal and social issue makes sense, the problem occurs when this dynamic becomes over-generalized so that every student and group is seen to be a victim of traumatic violence and assault: "this discussion foregrounds concerns that protecting or helping students might actually coddle them, stunting their growth into mature, well-adjusted adults who contribute the health of American democracy. Educators also fear that coddling could endanger the professional standing of instructors and, ultimately, intellectual freedom, as it compels instructors to accommodate even the slightest student sensitivity" (57).

Once again, the issue is that this well-intentioned pedagogy may end up harming students, teachers, and the educational process, and a central problem is that it is hard to determine how to respond to each student's particular needs, while at the same time holding onto shared assessment criteria.[89]

As we have seen, one of the biggest challenges concerns what constitutes trauma and what should be considered only a form of mental discomfort: "Similarly, general stress and discomfort are not exactly the same as traumatic stress. Drawing on the *Diagnostic and Statistical Manual*, clinician Abigail Powers Lott defines traumatic stress as stemming from direct or indirect exposure to actual or threatened death, serious injury, or sexual violence through 'terrible events' that are generally outside the range of daily human experience [and] are emotionally painful, intense, and distressing'" (59). At times, Day appears to argue that every student has been traumatized, but at other times, she applies a very narrow definition related to PTSD. A possible reason for this contradiction is that people are equating stress and unhappiness with the experience of actual violence. In fact, the concept of symbolic violence opens the door for an expansive notion of trauma.[90]

Since most of the teachers have little understanding of psychopathology, they tend to combine together very different diagnostic categories and symptoms:

> Thus, when authors equate triggering with discomfort, curling up in a ball and sobbing (Essig), or personal frailty (Jarvie), they oversimplify and misrepresent trauma responses and portray trauma survivors as over-sensitive and weak, needing a push in the direction of emotional maturity, rather than viewing them as already resilient. Clearly, to describe traumatic stress and triggering simply as discomfort would be inaccurate.
>
> (60)

Even though Day argues here that we should not equate discomfort with trauma, that is exactly what we find in many modes of trauma-informed pedagogy.

In an effort to distinguish mental discomfort from real trauma, Day falls back on a simple opposition that is not based on a clear understanding of unconscious defense mechanisms:

> Discomfort appears within the normal range of human experiences and human capacity for processing difficult experiences and material. Indeed, as many instructors have noted, discomfort may even be a necessary precursor to meaningful learning. Traumatic stress, on the other hand, presents an obstacle to learning and can possibly cause long-term negative impacts on an individual's physical, psychological, emotional, social, and spiritual well-being.
>
> (60)

Using this distinction between discomfort and trauma, it is unclear how a teacher can know if students are suffering from mild stress or if their issues represent a long-term obstacle to learning.[91] From a psychoanalytic perspective, one of the determining factors is the issue of how the expression of suffering is being used to gain a sense of identity or to affect other people. Moreover, if one acknowledges that this representation of suffering and trauma can be unconscious, then it is necessary to see how a person can engage in self-deception.[92] Since psychoanalysis is often repressed in these discussions, the result is that a naïve sense of student subjectivity is employed.

For Freud, a true traumatic response entails the suspension of the pleasure principle and a lack of anxiety and symbolization in relation to an unexpected event.[93] Since the memory of the trauma has not been symbolized, it returns to the real in the form of a perception. This type of traumatic experience is not very common, and it has little to do with the hysterical use of suffering, which is often related to imaginary fantasies and repressed desires and fears.[94] Furthermore, in the case of phobias and other anxiety-related neuroses, the main factor deals with how a real cause for concern is displaced onto a symbolic substitute.[95] Once again, we are not talking about an event that returns to the mind in the form of an unsymbolized reality; instead, with panic attacks, it is the symbolic substitution and displacement that triggers an inappropriate reflexive response.[96]

Due to the lack of understanding concerning the difference between hysterical symptoms of distress and the return of traumatic memories in the real, educators and therapists tend to hold onto a contradictory notion of trauma itself:

> Another misunderstanding circulated by the trigger warning debates is the notion that trauma is good and benefits education. Essig, for example, claims that learning is not only painful, but "ugly and traumatic," and that "real education" requires these things (par. 8; 11). Such assertions appear to function on imprecise and largely unproductive definitions of trauma. The popular notion that "learning itself is traumatic" equates trauma with an existential kind of pain. That is, education is traumatic for students because it causes them to come face-to-face with uncomfortable truths and to undergo transformation in the process, a transformation that is emotionally painful but ultimately beneficial.
>
> (62)

While Freud did argue that learning is often accompanied by unpleasure, his main point was that pleasure involves an effort to escape from reality.[97] With this theory in mind, it makes no sense to argue for a mode of education that involves no discomfort, but this does not mean that one should try to purposely trigger students.

Even though Day herself tends to over-generalize about the number of students who suffer from PTSD, she does at times realize that the exaggeration of trauma can function to hide real traumatic causes as more subtle forms of discomfort gain all of the attention:

> composition literature privileges perspectives on trauma as existential crisis or as a metaphor for transformation, but this definition belittles literal traumatic experiences by equating them with routine challenges. This inaccuracy is made

clear by comparison with clinical definitions. SAMHSA defines trauma as experiences, events, or circumstances that cause intense physical and psychological stress reactions by threatening physical and/or emotional harm (*TIP 57* xix)
(62–63)

The main problem with this definition of trauma is that the meaning of emotional harm is very vague and can relate to a whole series of different responses.[98]

A possible cause for this unclear definition of trauma is that activists seeking accommodations for students with different mental issues tend to attack any attempt to establish clear boundaries between the rational and the emotional:

> For instance, drawing on Margaret Price's *Mad At School*, Carter argues that, even though higher education has made great strides toward accommodation and inclusion for those dealing with mental illness/disability – which can sometimes result from/in trauma – there remains a tenacious though implicit notion that mental illness/disability and associated emotional responses are contrary to the "rational realm" of the classroom, and "crazy" students are thus referred outside the classroom to external resources (e.g. counseling centers, disability offices, tutoring centers) but their unique perspectives are not simultaneously welcome.
>
> (64)

This desire to protect students with disabilities and illnesses has resulted in a situation where it becomes politically incorrect to try to argue for the teaching of reason or the distinction between rationality and irrationality.[99] In trying to protect students with clear mental issues, institutions of higher education have undermined their own foundational principles. Perhaps a reason for this problem is the notion that every young person should go to college, and if these people have severe psychological or physical issues, the schools have to accommodate their specific needs. Instead of students getting help from outside sources, the idea is that universities and colleges need to provide psychological services for every person.[100] Not only does this ideology result in spending a great deal of money on non-educational activities, but it also calls into question the ability to teach reason and the scientific method in an equal manner.

An essential problem facing contemporary universities and colleges is that it is unclear what they should really be doing. Are they centers of research and instruction, or are they places where social and psychological problems are resolved?[101] Another related issue concerns the desire to accept and educate every student – even if the students do not have the mental or physical ability to learn the material.[102] As Day indicates, students who do suffer from serious mental issues have a high drop-out rate, and this is during a period where unprecedented accommodations are being made: "the persistent stigma surrounding mental illness/disability and trauma responses excludes such students from meaningful membership in classroom communities and contributes to drop-out rates of 56.1% for students with "mental illness" and 23.6% for students 'serious emotional disturbance'" (64). Day appears to argue that the reason why these students are dropping out of college is because they are being stigmatized, but the real reason may be that they are unable to do the work.[103]

Since we know that, on average, people who earn college degrees make more money and have better life outcomes, it does seem to be discriminatory to prevent specific types of people from attending these institutions, but if they are unable to do the work in an effective manner, then it is unclear how anyone is helped by simply accommodating students.[104] A bigger issue is the notion that universities are supposed to heal all social ills and inequalities when the reality is that these schools, on average, actually enhance inequality and reduce social mobility.[105] The reason for this problem is not that they are not helping students who need special attention. The real issue is that selective admission policies enhance pre-existing social hierarchies. As I argue in my book *Educating Inequality*, we cannot expect these schools to make society more just and fair, and when we ask them to heal all personal and social conflicts, they end up ignoring their basic function of using reason to discover and communicate truth through shared methods and empirical testing. These institutions also have a crucial role in verifying expertise and replacing the old aristocratic model with a meritocratic system.

Although the very idea of a meritocracy has come under attack, a modern liberal democracy relies on an accurate assessment of people's abilities and knowledge.[106] If we find that these institutions fail to pursue their core mission, the response should not be simply to reject their main values and practices; instead, we need to find ways to protect reason and impartial judgment. Unfortunately, when schools define students as being victims of trauma who need to be treated by teachers for their particular issues, reason is replaced by emotion, and special accommodation substitutes for equal treatment.[107] Although Day at times seeks to clearly distinguish between students who are really suffering from PTSD and those who have other mental issues, she ends up claiming that most students have been traumatized: "it assumes traumatic stress is an atypical student experience that requires only occasional accommodation, even though studies show that the majority of college students have experienced trauma, particularly females and racial minorities" (65). Like so many other promoters of trauma-informed pedagogy, Day alternates between over-generalizing about trauma and seeking a clear distinction between trauma and mental discomfort. This desire to affirm opposite positions reflects a contradictory perspective, which tries to combine scientific reason with an emotional commitment to a specific educational ideology. One cannot say at the same time that most students suffer from PTSD, and it is a very rare condition.[108]

It is also contradictory to posit that students are resilient, but they need special attention and care: "it stigmatizes survivors as atypical members of classroom communities whose inability to emotionally regulate might get 'in the way' of other students' learning, rather than treating them as resilient individuals whose perspectives might enrich all students' classroom experiences" (65). Once again, we have to ask if students are being represented as being highly resilient, or are they being seen as highly vulnerable and needing special care?[109] Instead of resolving this contradiction, Day pivots and turns her focus to the issue of student academic freedom: "The debate over trigger warnings and safe spaces thus brings instructors' academic or intellectual freedom to the forefront while largely ignoring *students'* right to intellectual freedom" (66). In turning the issue of trigger warnings and other academic accommodations into a question of student academic freedom, Day feeds a misguided notion of the roles of students and teachers in higher education. Instead of defending expertise and reason, the focus on the student feeds the cult of the amateur in contemporary politics and culture.[110] Thus, one cause for the Right-wing attack on universities, reason, and expertise is the argument that teachers do not have any special role in the production and dissemination of knowledge.[111] Rather than the promotion of the teacher's academic freedom, we now have a desire to protect a student's ability to say and do whatever they want.[112] This false representation of academic freedom eliminates the focus on pursuing truth wherever it leads through the use of shared concepts, theories, and methods; instead, every opinion and ideology is supposed to be valued equally.

A central problem facing higher education, then, is not only are universities and colleges expected to resolve the students' mental health issues, but an expanded notion of trauma threatens to represent every student as a vulnerable victim. In response to this promotion of a hysterical form of subjectivity, teachers are asked to act as therapists – even though they have little training. Due in part to the repression of psychoanalysis inside and outside of higher education, false modes of therapy are applied as teachers and other adults feed their narcissism by taking on the position of the ones who know and care. While knowing and caring should be a good thing, when they are motivated by unconscious desires and defense mechanisms, they can be highly destructive. As we shall see in the next chapter, when the idealizing transference is not analyzed, it can create a type of dependency and mind-control that we often find in CBT and other forms of therapy based on suggestion and the quick resolution of complex mental issues.

Notes

1 Harrison, Neil, Jacqueline Burke, and Ivan Clarke. "Risky teaching: Developing a trauma-informed pedagogy for higher education." *Teaching in Higher Education* 28.1 (2023): 180–194.
2 Day, Michelle. *Wounds and Writing: Building Trauma-Informed Approaches to Writing Pedagogy.* PhD dissertation. University of Louisville, 2019.
3 Pinker, Steven. "Enlightenment now, the case for reason, science, humanism, and progress." *Revista Española de Investigaciones Sociológicas (REIS)* 170.170 (2020): 163–167.
4 Pinker, Steven. *The Better Angels of Our Nature: Why Violence Has Declined.* Penguin Books, 2012.
5 Bryant, Richard A. "Post-traumatic stress disorder: A state-of-the-art review of evidence and challenges." *World Psychiatry* 18.3 (2019): 259–269.
6 May, Casey L., and Blair E. Wisco. "Defining trauma: How level of exposure and proximity affect risk for posttraumatic stress disorder." *Psychological Trauma: Theory, Research, Practice, and Policy* 8.2 (2016): 233.

7 Myta, Alexa. *Teacher Perceptions of Trauma: How Teacher Empathy and Experienced Adversity Aid in Recognizing Trauma in the Classroom.* Diss. William James College, 2021.

8 Zembylas, Michalinos. "The politics of trauma: Empathy, reconciliation and peace education." *Journal of Peace Education* 4.2 (2007): 207–224.

9 Freud, Sigmund. *Civilization and Its Discontents.* Broadview Press, 2015.

10 Garcia, Emanuel E. "Freud's seduction theory." *The Psychoanalytic Study of the Child* 42.1 (1987): 443–468.

11 Cohen, Jonathan. "Trauma and repression." *Psychoanalytic Inquiry* 5.1 (1985): 163–189.

12 Katz, Jay. "On primary gain and secondary gain." *The Psychoanalytic Study of the Child* 18.1 (1963): 9–50.

13 Samuels, Robert, and Robert Samuels. "Pathos, Hysteria, and the left." *Zizek and the Rhetorical Unconscious: Global Politics, Philosophy, and Subjectivity.* Springer Nature, 2020, 33–47.

14 Cole, Alyson Manda. *The Cult of True Victimhood: From the War on Welfare to the War on Terror.* Stanford University Press, 2007.

15 Freud, Sigmund. *Dora: An Analysis of a Case of Hysteria.* Simon and Schuster, 1997.

16 Jacoby, Tami Amanda. "A theory of victimhood: Politics, conflict and the construction of victim-based identity." *Millennium* 43.2 (2015): 511–530.

17 Freud, Sigmund. *Group Psychology and the Analysis of the Ego.* WW Norton & Company, 1975.

18 Breithaupt, Fritz. *The Dark Sides of Empathy.* Cornell University Press, 2019.

19 Freud, Sigmund. "Project for a scientific psychology. Standard Edition, vol. 1." *Hogarth Press, London* 1958 (1895): 295–397.

20 Lacan, Jacques. *Seminar XI: The Four Fundamental Concepts of Psychoanalysis.* Trans. Alan Sheridan. New York, London: Norton & Company, 1977.

21 Freud, Sigmund. "The dynamics of transference." *Classics in Psychoanalytic Techniques* 12 (1912): 97–108.

22 Jackson, Donald D., and Jay Haley. "Transference revisited." *The Journal of Nervous and Mental Disease* 137.4 (1963): 363–371.

23 Gildersleeve, Matthew. "Demystifying complexes, transference, and narcissistic personality disorder with Jung and Lacan." *Indian Journal of Psychological Medicine* 38.3 (2016): 269–272.

24 Stone, Alison. *Feminism, Psychoanalysis, and Maternal Subjectivity.* Routledge, 2013.

25 Samuels, Robert. "(Liberal) narcissism." *Routledge Handbook of Psychoanalytic Political Theory.* Routledge, 2019, 151–161.

26 Samuels, Robert. *(Mis) Understanding Freud with Lacan, Zizek, and Neuroscience.* Springer Nature, 2022.

27 Freud, Sigmund, et al. *Psycho-Analysis and the War Neuroses.* DigiCat, 2022.

28 Freud, Sigmund. "The history of the psychoanalytic movement." *The Psychoanalytic Review (1913–1957)* 3 (1916): 406.

29 Freud, Sigmund. "Remembering, repeating and working-through (Further recommendations on the technique of psycho-analysis II)." *The Standard Edition of the Complete Psychological Works of Sigmund Freud. Vol. XII: (1911–1913).* Routledge, 1914.

30 Freud, Sigmund, and Joseph Breuer. *Studies in Hysteria.* Penguin, 2004.

31 Spence, Sean A. "Hysteria: A new look." *Psychiatry* 5.2 (2006): 56–60.

32 Van der Kolk, Bessel A. "Trauma, neuroscience, and the etiology of hysteria: An exploration of the relevance of Breuer and Freud's 1893 article in light of modern science." *Journal of the American Academy of Psychoanalysis* 28.2 (2000): 237–262.

33 Bistoen, Gregory, and Gregory Bistoen. "The Lacanian concept of the real and the psychoanalytical take on trauma." *Trauma, Ethics and the Political Beyond PTSD: The Dislocations of the Real.* Springer, 2016, 53–82.

34   Artime, Tiffany M., Katherine R. Buchholz, and Matthew Jakupcak. "Mental health symptoms and treatment utilization among trauma-exposed college students." *Psychological Trauma: Theory, Research, Practice, and Policy* 11.3 (2019): 274.

35   Read, Jennifer P., et al. "PTSD symptom course during the first year of college." *Psychological Trauma: Theory, Research, Practice, and Policy* 8.3 (2016): 393.

36   Stein, Dan J., et al. "Post-traumatic stress disorder: Medicine and politics." *The Lancet* 369.9556 (2007): 139–144.

37   Stein, Dan J., et al. "Post-traumatic stress disorder: Medicine and politics." *The Lancet* 369.9556 (2007): 139–144.

38   Pollock, Griselda. "Art/trauma/representation." *Parallax* 15.1 (2009): 40–54.

39   Rickert, Thomas Joseph. *Acts of Enjoyment: Rhetoric, Žižek, and the Return of the Subject.* University of Pittsburgh Press, 2007.

40   Bracher, Mark. *The Writing Cure: Psychoanalysis, Composition, and the Aims of Education.* SIU Press, 1999.

41   Samuels, Robert. *Teaching Writing, Rhetoric, and Reason at the Globalizing University.* Routledge, 2020.

42   Orgad, Shani. "The survivor in contemporary culture and public discourse: A genealogy." *The Communication Review* 12.2 (2009): 132–161.

43   Berman, Jeffrey. "The Teaching Cure." *Psychoanalysis and Narrative Medicine*, SUNY Press, 2008, 229.

44   Berman, Jeffrey. "The talking cure and the writing cure." *Philosophy, Psychiatry, & Psychology* 17.3 (2010): 255–257.

45   Fish, Stanley. *Save the World on Your Own Time.* Oxford University Press, 2008.

46   Haines, Staci K. *The Politics of Trauma: Somatics, Healing, and Social Justice.* North Atlantic Books, 2019.

47   Knight, Carolyn. "Trauma-informed social work practice: Practice considerations and challenges." *Clinical Social Work Journal* 43 (2015): 25–37.

48   Schore, Judith R., and Allan N. Schore. "Clinical social work and regulation theory: Implications of neurobiological models of attachment." *Adult Attachment in Clinical Social Work: Practice, Research, and Policy.* Springer, 2011, 57–75.

49   Samuels, Robert. *Freud for the Twenty-First Century: The Science of Everyday Life.* Springer, 2019.

50   Moses, Ira. "The misuse of empathy in psychoanalysis." *Contemporary Psychoanalysis* 24.4 (1988): 577–594.

51   Elliott, Robert, et al. "Empathy." *Psychotherapy* 48.1 (2011): 43.

52   Hassan, Steven A., and M. J. Shah. "The anatomy of undue influence used by terrorist cults and traffickers to induce helplessness and trauma, so creating false identities." *Ethics, Medicine and Public Health* 8 (2019): 97–107.

53   Freud, Sigmund. *Group Psychology and the Analysis of the Ego.* WW Norton & Company, 1975.

54   Smith, Tawnya D. "Teaching through trauma: Compassion fatigue, burnout, or secondary traumatic stress?." *Trauma and Resilience in Music Education.* Routledge, 2021, 49–63.

55   Zembylas, Michalinos. "Beyond teacher cognition and teacher beliefs: The value of the ethnography of emotions in teaching." *International Journal of Qualitative Studies in Education* 18.4 (2005): 465–487.

56   Carello, Janice, and Lisa D. Butler. "Practicing what we teach: Trauma-informed educational practice." *Journal of Teaching in Social Work* 35.3 (2015): 262–278.

57   Moysiuk, Julie. "A critique of diversity, inclusion and equity policies in Canadian universities." *Political Science Undergraduate Review* 4.1 (2019): 65–71.

58   Brunzell, Tom, Helen Stokes, and Lea Waters. "Shifting teacher practice in trauma-affected classrooms: Practice pedagogy strategies within a trauma-informed positive education model." *School Mental Health* 11.3 (2019): 600–614.

59 Inoue, Asao B. *Above the Well: An Antiracist Literacy Argument from a Boy of Color*. University Press of Colorado, 2021.

60 Bailes, Jonathan Richard. *Consciousness and the Limits of Social Conformity: A Theory of Ideology Through the Works of Marcuse, Jameson and Žižek*. Diss. UCL. University College London, 2017.

61 Bailes, Jonathan Richard. *Consciousness and the Limits of Social Conformity: A Theory of Ideology Through the Works of Marcuse, Jameson and Žižek*. Diss. UCL. University College London, 2017.

62 Samuels, Robert. *Teaching the Rhetoric of Resistance: The Popular Holocaust and Social Change in a Post-9/11 World*. Springer, 2007.

63 Freud's, In. "Negation." *Standard Edition* 19 (2022).

64 Donlevy, J. Kent, Dianne Gereluk, and Jim Brandon. "Trigger warnings, freedom of speech, and academic freedom in higher education." *Education & Law Journal* 28.1 (2018): 1–41.

65 Kitrosser, Heidi. "Free speech, higher education, and the PC narrative." *Minnesota Law Review* 101 (2016): 1987.

66 Cullinan, John, Sharon Walsh, and Darragh Flannery. "Socioeconomic disparities in unmet need for student mental health services in higher education." *Applied Health Economics and Health Policy* 18 (2020): 223–235.

67 Borman, Geoffrey D., and Steven M. Kimball. "Teacher quality and educational equality: Do teachers with higher standards-based evaluation ratings close student achievement gaps?" *The Elementary School Journal* 106.1 (2005): 3–20.

68 Brunzell, Tom, Lea Waters, and Helen Stokes. "Teaching with strengths in trauma-affected students: A new approach to healing and growth in the classroom." *American Journal of Orthopsychiatry* 85.1 (2015): 3.

69 Hill, Vikki, et al. "Belonging through assessment: Pipelines of compassion QAA Collaborative Enhancement Project 2021." UAL, University of Arts London, 2023.

70 Gottfredson, Nisha C., et al. "Does diversity at undergraduate institutions influence student outcomes?" *Journal of Diversity in Higher Education* 1.2 (2008): 80.

71 Bloom, Diane S., et al. "Are my students like me? The path to color-blindness and white racial identity development." *Education and Urban Society* 47.5 (2015): 555–575.

72 Peters, Terri, et al. "What's race got to do with it?: Preservice teachers and white racial identity." *Current Issues in Education* 19.1 (2016).

73 Steinmetz, Carl H. D. "Criticism of the concepts of diversity and inclusion in Western countries." *Advances in Social Sciences Research Journal* 8.9 (2021): 116–132.

74 Ballard, Dawna, et al. "When words do not matter: Identifying actions to effect diversity, equity, and inclusion in the academy." *Management Communication Quarterly* 34.4 (2020): 590–616.

75 Samuels, Robert, and Robert Samuels. "Pathos, Hysteria, and the left." *Zizek and the Rhetorical Unconscious: Global Politics, Philosophy, and Subjectivity*. Springer, 2020, 33–47.

76 Horowitz, Mark, Anthony L. Haynor, and Kenneth Kickham. "'Undeserved' grades or 'underserved' students? Faculty anxieties and eroding standards in the corporate university." *Higher Education Politics & Economics* 9.1 (2023): 44–83.

77 Wilson, Kristen Nicole. *The Impact of Mental Health and Trauma on Student Retention: A Faculty Perspective*. Wilmington University (Delaware), 2023.

78 Heller, Janet Ruth. "Contingent faculty and the evaluation process." *College Composition and Communication* 64.1 (2012): A8–A12.

79 Trout, Paul. "Deconstructing an evaluation form." *The Montana Professor* 8.3 (1998).

80 Samuels, Bob. "Contingent faculty and academic freedom in the age of Trump: Organizing the disenfranchised is the key to success." *FORUM: Issues about Part-Time and Contingent Faculty*. Vol. 21. No. 2. NCTE, 2018.

81 Weis, Robert, and Sophie A. Bittner. "College students' access to academic accommodations over time: Evidence of a Matthew effect in higher education." *Psychological Injury and Law* 15.3 (2022): 236–252.

82 Vance, Lisa L., and Katherine C. Aquino. "Dealing with the impact of long COVID on college campuses." *Disability Compliance for Higher Education* 28.7 (2023): 6–7.

83 Schott, Robin May. " 'Not just victims . . . but': Toward a critical theory of the victim." *Women and Violence: The Agency of Victims and Perpetrators*. London: Palgrave Macmillan UK, 2015, 178–194.

84 Carello, Janice, and Lisa D. Butler. "Potentially perilous pedagogies: Teaching trauma is not the same as trauma-informed teaching." *Journal of Trauma & Dissociation* 15.2 (2014): 153–168.

85 Cook, Joan M., Elana Newman, and Vanessa Simiola. "Trauma training: Competencies, initiatives, and resources." *Psychotherapy* 56.3 (2019): 409.

86 Noel, Hans. "Ideological factions in the republican and democratic parties." *The ANNALS of the American Academy of Political and Social Science* 667.1 (2016): 166–188.

87 Freeman, Tabitha. "Psychoanalytic concepts of fatherhood: Patriarchal paradoxes and the presence of an absent authority." *Studies in Gender and Sexuality* 9.2 (2008): 113–139.

88 Kimble, Matthew, et al. "Trauma-specific reactions to sexual assault content in college students: Considerations for content warnings." *Human Arenas* (2023): 1–18.

89 Hill, V., Broadhead, S., Bunting, L., da Costa, L., Currant, N., Greated, M., . . . & Stevens, T. *Belonging through Assessment: Pipelines of Compassion QAA Collaborative Enhancement Project 2021*, University of Arts London, 2023.

90 Bachner, Sally. "The wrong victims: Terrorism, trauma, and symbolic violence." *Interventions: Activists and Academics Respond to Violence*. New York: Palgrave Macmillan US, 2004, 23–28.

91 Rothbaum, Barbara Olasov, and Michael Davis. "Applying learning principles to the treatment of post-trauma reactions." *Annals of the New York Academy of Sciences* 1008.1 (2003): 112–121.

92 Joseph, Rhawn. "Awareness, the origin of thought, and the role of conscious self-deception in resistance and repression." *Psychological Reports* 46.3 (1980): 767–781.

93 Freud, Sigmund. *Beyond the Pleasure Principle*. Penguin UK, 2003.

94 Freud, Sigmund. *Five Lectures on Psychoanalysis*. WW Norton & Company, 1977.

95 Freud, Sigmund. *Obsessions and Phobias*. Read Books Ltd, 2014.

96 Masi, Franco. "The psychodynamic of panic attacks: A useful integration of psychoanalysis and neuroscience." *The International Journal of Psychoanalysis* 85.2 (2004): 311–336.

97 Samuels, Robert, and Robert Samuels. "The pleasure principle and the death drive." *Freud for the Twenty-First Century: The Science of Everyday Life*. Springer, 2019, 17–25.

98 Weathers, Frank W., and Terence M. Keane. "The criterion a problem revisited: Controversies and challenges in defining and measuring psychological trauma." *Journal of Traumatic Stress* 20.2 (2007): 107–121.

99 Carter, Angela M. "When silence said everything: Reconceptualizing trauma through critical disability studies." *Lateral* 10.1 (2021).

100 Watkins, Daphne C., Justin B. Hunt, and Daniel Eisenberg. "Increased demand for mental health services on college campuses: Perspectives from administrators." *Qualitative Social Work* 11.3 (2012): 319–337.

101 Gonzales, Leslie D. "Responding to mission creep: Faculty members as cosmopolitan agents." *Higher Education* 64 (2012): 337–353.

102 Karabel, Jerome. "Open admissions: Toward meritocracy or democracy?" *Change: The Magazine of Higher Learning* 4.4 (1972): 38–43.
103 Tamin, S. K. "Relevance of mental health issues in university student dropouts." *Occupational Medicine* 63.6 (2013): 410–414.
104 Baum, Sandy. "Higher education earnings premium: Value, variation, and trends." *Urban Institute.* February, 2014.
105 Samuels, Robert. *Educating Inequality: Beyond the Political Myths of Higher Education and the Job Market.* Routledge, 2017.
106 Meroe, Aundra Saa. "Democracy, meritocracy and the uses of education." *Journal of Negro Education* 83.4 (2014): 485–498.
107 Hernandez, Danny. *Students with Disabiltiies and Identity Development: Higher Education, Ableism, Meritocracy, and Meaning Making.* Diss. University of Southern California, 2021.
108 Read, Jennifer P., et al. "Rates of DSM–IV–TR trauma exposure and posttraumatic stress disorder among newly matriculated college students." *Psychological Trauma: Theory, Research, Practice, and Policy* 3.2 (2011): 148.
109 Wall, Carrie R. Giboney. "Relationship over reproach: Fostering resilience by embracing a trauma-informed approach to elementary education." *Journal of Aggression, Maltreatment & Trauma* 30.1 (2021): 118–137.
110 Keen, Andrew, and Magnus Ramage. "The cult of the amateur." *Online Communication and Collaboration: A Reader.* Routledge, 2010, 251–255.
111 Grundmann, Reiner. "The rightful place of expertise." *Questioning Experts and Expertise.* Routledge, 2022, 18–32.
112 Macfarlane, Bruce. *Freedom to Learn: The Threat to Student Academic Freedom and Why It Needs to Be Reclaimed.* Routledge, 2016.

Chapter 4

Coddling Trauma

The Center-Right Turns to CBT

This chapter looks at how politics has helped to shape how we think about student mental health, trauma, and the role of higher education in responding to the mental suffering of students. In examining Greg Lukianoff's and Jonathan Haidt's *The Coddling of the American Mind*, we discover that social perceptions of student mental health issues have been affected by a center-Right ideology combining together conservative morality with a backlash against Left-wing politics and educational activism.[1] Furthermore, the proposed solution, CBT, represents a repression of psychoanalysis and a new form of hypnotic mind-control. Through the combination of premodern moralism and libertarian capitalism, a false form of liberalism is presented, and one of the results is that hysteria and narcissism continue to be reinforced and misunderstood.

The Causes of Our Discontent

According to Lukianoff and Haidt, there are three main untruths that are shaping our culture and undermining higher education and the mental health of young adults: "The Untruth of Fragility: What doesn't kill you makes you weaker. The Untruth of Emotional Reasoning: Always trust your feelings. The Untruth of Us Versus Them: Life is a battle between good people and evil people" (4–5). What these authors are arguing is that our society is shaped by a series of false premises concerning emotions, mental suffering, and binary thinking. Although their main focus appears to be the replacement of reason with emotion in higher education, their version of tough love draws from a combination of conservative morality and modern psychology: "While many propositions are untrue, in order to be classified as a Great Untruth, an idea must meet three criteria: It contradicts ancient wisdom (ideas found widely in the wisdom literatures of many cultures). It contradicts modern psychological research on well-being. It harms the individuals and communities who embrace it" (4). One thing to point out about this use of both ancient wisdom and modern psychology is that it allows for the conjuring of science to justify traditional beliefs.[2]

DOI: 10.4324/9781003545668-4

Lukianoff and Haidt focus on how young adults are reporting higher levels of anxiety and depression at a time when they have more access to mental health practitioners:

> To name just a few of these problems: Teen anxiety, depression, and suicide rates have risen sharply in the last few years. The culture on many college campuses has become more ideologically uniform, compromising the ability of scholars to seek truth, and of students to learn from a broad range of thinkers. Extremists have proliferated on the far right and the far left, provoking one another to ever deeper levels of hatred. Social media has channeled partisan passions into the creation of a 'callout culture'; anyone can be publicly shamed for saying something well-intentioned that someone else interprets uncharitably. New-media platforms and outlets allow citizens to retreat into self-confirmatory bubbles, where their worst fears about the evils of the other side can be confirmed and amplified by extremists and cyber trolls intent on sowing discord and division.
>
> (5)

There are several different issues brought up in the passage, but the main underlying idea is that as our culture has become more polarized and extreme, young adults are complaining more about their mental health, and a leading cause for all of these factors is that people are being censored for their partisan beliefs.[3] In other words, a culture war is harming young adults' mental health, but the real issue is that people have become overly sensitive to ideas and speech that differ from their own ideology.

The reason why these authors want to combine a concern for student mental health with an analysis of cancel culture is that they desire to attack both supposed Left-wing indoctrination in higher education and the catering to students' feelings:

> In years past, administrators were motivated to create campus speech codes in order to curtail what they deemed to be racist or sexist speech. Increasingly, however, the rationale for speech codes and speaker disinvitations was becoming medicalized: Students claimed that certain kinds of speech – and even the content of some books and courses – interfered with their ability to function. They wanted protection from material that they believed could jeopardize their mental health by "triggering" them, or making them "feel unsafe."
>
> (6)

According to Lukianoff and Haidt, university students should be exposed to a variety of viewpoints, but academic freedom is being curtailed because faculty and administrators are afraid to upset students by presenting ideas that may make them feel bad or traumatized.[4] What they do not say is that free speech has been weaponized by the Right in order to attack the perceived Left-wing bias of higher education.[5] From this backlash perspective, trauma-informed pedagogy and the desire to protect students from triggering content is a political project dedicated to censoring conservatives and the Right.[6]

What really upsets these scholars is not that the pure pursuit of truth through reason and the scientific method is being undermined. What they are really countering is the push to protect minoritized students against material that they find marginalizes their own identity: "However, in 2015, four Columbia undergraduates wrote an essay in the school newspaper arguing that students 'need to feel safe in the classroom' but 'many texts in the Western canon' are 'wrought with histories and narratives of exclusion and oppression' and contain 'triggering and offensive material that marginalizes student identities in the classroom" (6). Although Lukianoff and Haidt insist that they are protecting academic freedom for everyone, most of their examples deal with programs and policies focused on creating a safe space for under-represented minority students.[7]

Driving this discourse is thus a Right-wing backlash against minority-based social movements, and even when they lament the fact that students, in general, are afraid to encounter ideas that challenge their own ideologies, what they end up doing, knowingly or unknowingly, is to posit that students should be exposed to racist, sexist, and homophobic speech.[8] Although it is common to think that modern reason and education is centered on total free speech, the reality is that higher education should be based on truth and science and not on political ideologies and opinions.[9]

One reason why it is important to reveal the underlying politics of Lukianoff's and Haidt's approach is that it is vital to distinguish between the college mental health crisis and the broader culture war.[10] On the level of student mental health, I have stressed how a mode of student hysteria is being accommodated by a narcissistic form of therapy, but this dynamic is different from the Right-wing complaint that conservative and libertarian students and faculty are being censored because it hurts the feelings and beliefs of Left-wing students and professors.[11] By trying to frame these issues in the context of a polarized culture war, the focus moves from problems concerning mental health to ones dealing with politics. Moreover, even though Lukianoff and Haidt see polarization as a major untruth, they engage in this type of thinking throughout their work.

CBT and the Repression of Psychoanalysis

Interestingly, these authors believe that even when students do not think that they will be harmed by hearing upsetting speech, some students fear that other students will be harmed: "What is new today is the premise that students are fragile. Even those who are not fragile themselves often believe that others are in danger and therefore need protection. There is no expectation that students will grow stronger from their encounters with speech or texts they label 'triggering'" (7). The main idea here is that students should be exposed to upsetting material because it will make them stronger and less fragile.[12] In applying ideas from Cognitive Behavioral Therapy (CBT), they posit that exposure reduces fear and anxiety, which are themselves caused by faulty thinking: "CBT teaches you to notice when you are engaging in various "cognitive distortions," such as "catastrophizing" (If I fail this quiz, I'll fail the class and be kicked out of school, and then I'll never get a job . . .) and "negative filtering" (only paying attention to negative feedback instead of noticing praise as well). These distorted and irrational thought patterns are hallmarks of depression and anxiety disorders" (8). This turn to CBT not only represses psychoanalysis but also relies on a form of mind-control dedicated to getting patients to accept the suggestions of the idealized authority (the therapist).[13] Therefore, instead of working through the transference through the use of free association and analytic neutrality, this method returns to the pre-psychoanalytic use of direct and indirect hypnosis.[14]

In repressing the psychoanalytic concepts of the unconscious, transference, neutrality, free association, hysteria, and narcissism, CBT represents a fast but ineffective way of trying to change people's thoughts by replacing them with the ideas of the therapist.[15] Since Lukianoff and Haidt believe that students have been indoctrinated by a Left-wing ideology that makes them fragile and hyper-sensitive, their solution is to subject them to a new, more adaptive ideology:

> Their beliefs about their own and others' fragility in the face of ideas they dislike would become self-fulfilling prophecies. Not only would students come to believe that they can't handle such things, but if they acted on that belief and avoided exposure, eventually they would become less able to do so. If students succeeded in creating bubbles of intellectual "safety" in college, they would set themselves up for even greater anxiety and conflict after graduation, when they will certainly encounter many more people with more extreme views.
>
> (9)

According to this approach, students, thus, need to grow comfortable with encountering extreme ideologies, and the best place to expose them to these views is in college. Yet, we must ask why college is supposed to play this therapeutic role, and is it a good thing to become tolerant of intolerance?[16]

From the perspective of CBT, all of these issues come down to people having distorted thoughts, which can be changed through exposure or suggestion: "Many university students are learning to think in distorted ways, and this increases their likelihood of becoming fragile, anxious, and easily hurt" (9). On one level, it is correct to say that these mental health issues derive from thoughts, but we have to examine where these thoughts come from and how they are best dealt with. If a therapist simply tries to tell a patient to think different thoughts, the patient will become dependent on the therapist, and the real cause for these faulty ideas will never be discovered.[17] In fact, one reason why Freud gave up hypnosis is that he found that it only gave temporary relief, and old symptoms would usually return.[18] Freud also did not think that patients should become dependent on an idealized authority because idealization is based on the suspension of reality testing.[19]

As a way of demonizing education, which is a common Right-wing move, Luki-anoff and Haidt argue that students are internalizing self-destructive attitudes they are learning them from their teachers and parents:

> we argued that many parents, K-12 teachers, professors, and university admin-istrators have been unknowingly teaching a generation of students to engage in the mental habits commonly seen in people who suffer from anxiety and depres-sion. We suggested that students were beginning to react to words, books, and visiting speakers with fear and anger because they had been taught to exagger-ate danger, use dichotomous (or binary) thinking, amplify their first emotional responses, and engage in a number of other cognitive distortions.
>
> (10)

According to this mode of CBT-driven politics, the problem is that parents, teach-ers, and administrators have trained young people to focus on negative emotions and fear, and so what we need is a counter-form of mind-control.[20] While I have also warned against the way parents and teachers can have this harmful effect by rewarding and affirming the expression of negative emotions, I have argued that this trend is largely driven by narcissism and not Left-wing politics. Furthermore, the solution is not CBT or some form of exposure therapy; what we need is a greater understanding of psychoanalytic theory and practice.

Coddling the Culture War

What appears to really upset Lukianoff and Haidt is the fact that many conservative and Right-wing speakers have been criticized and canceled at American universi-ties because their speech has been deemed to be harmful to students:

> At some schools, a culture of defensive self-censorship seemed to be emerging, partly in response to students who were quick to "call out" or shame others for small things that they deemed to be insensitive – either to the student doing the calling out or to members of a group that the student was standing up for. We called this pattern vindictive protectiveness and argued that such behavior made it more difficult for all students to have open discussions in which they could practice the essential skills of critical thinking and civil disagreement.
>
> (11)

Although I do agree that a certain sector of the Left tends to use shame and other modes of indirect aggression to attack perceived opponents, the bigger issue is why are universities being charged with the responsibility of getting students not to be offended by offensive ideas?[21]

A possible reason for this emphasis on exposure to diverse viewpoints may relate to the perception by Republicans that they are not controlling the discourse at these institutions.[22] Moreover, there is a common confusion among the notions of viewpoint diversity, academic freedom, free speech, and the scientific method.[23] Since universities are founded on the principles of modern science, their main responsibility is to train people to take an impartial view of empirical evidence through the use of shared methods and theories. This process does not require tolerating everyone's opinions since people can have their own opinions but not their own facts.[24] In the effort to make these facts universal, the goal is to suspend bias and self-interest and not privilege particular ideologies – other than the ideology of modern reason. Lukianoff and Haidt may think that they are protecting reason by protecting the expression of every perspective, but the voicing of diverse ideologies does not lead to the truth; in fact, it most often leads to confusion and bias.

I have been arguing that Lukianoff's and Haidt's emphasis on student fragility and adult coddling is mostly a smokescreen for a political culture war that uses indirect discourse to recruit supporters of a particular, polarizing ideology.[25] For example, Lukianoff and Haidt turn to the issue of transgender rights and the use of pronouns to discuss the increased focus on emotions and safety in higher education:

> You can see the conflation of safety and feelings in another part of the memo, which urged faculty to use each student's preferred gender pronoun (for example, "zhe" or "they" for students who don't want to be referred to as "he" or "she"), not because this was respectful or appropriately sensitive but because a professor who uses an incorrect pronoun "prevents or impairs their safety in a classroom." If students have been told that they can request gender-neutral pronouns and then a professor fails to use one, students may be disappointed or upset. But are these students unsafe?
>
> (25)

Conservatives and the Right love to refer to the use of pronouns because they know that it will upset the people who believe that gender should only be based on biology in a strict binary opposition.[26] Although I am also concerned about the notion of overly protecting students and catering to their personal emotions, it is important not to confuse this concern with the political move to attack Democrats for seeking to protect transgender individuals.[27] Like so many other examples in their book, concerns about educational quality are used to score political points in a polarized culture war.

One of the favorite things for the Right to attack is the notion of racist microaggressions because it looks like minoritized subjects are simply being hyper-sensitive to minor comments:[28]

> A prime example of how some professors (and some administrators) encourage mental habits similar to the cognitive distortions is their promotion of the concept of "microaggressions," popularized in a 2007 article by Derald Wing Sue, a professor at Columbia University's Teachers College. Sue and several colleagues defined microaggressions as "brief and commonplace daily verbal, behavioral, or environmental indignities, whether intentional or unintentional,

that communicate hostile, derogatory, or negative racial slights and insults toward people of color." (The term was first applied to people of color but is now applied much more broadly.)

(40)

As Lukianoff and Haidt point out, microaggressions were first tied to the reactions of people of color to insults and slights that some might consider to be minor; even though their application has now been expanded, the criticism of microaggressions can be traced back to the Right-wing backlash against minority rights and the experiences of discrimination.[29] Since racism is now often presented in a more indirect and veiled manner, it is easier to dismiss claims of prejudice and discrimination, but what it is vital to understand is that what often drives the criticism of these responses by people of color is the insensitivity of the Right and their desire to not have their illiberal thoughts and feelings countered.[30] Since libertarians focus on their individual freedom, they do not feel that they should inhibit their aggression in order to placate others. As a way of reacting to perceived political correctness, the Right tends to celebrate free speech until it threatens their own identity.[31]

Although I do not think that Lukianoff and Haidt see themselves as Right-wing thinkers, many of their arguments feed this type of ideology. Not only do they make light of microaggressions and rationalize the allowance of hate speech, but they also tend to reinforce the Right-wing side of the culture war.[32] For instance, in their references to Herbert Marcuse, they follow the now-standard argument that this philosopher has helped to indoctrinate students into a mode of cultural Marxism, which justifies the censoring of conservative and Right-wing voices: "A 'truly 'liberating' tolerance," claimed Marcuse, is one that favors the weak and restrains the strong. Who are the weak and the strong? For Marcuse, writing in 1965, the weak was the political left and the strong was the political right" (65). Even though Lukianoff and Haidt claim that they are trying to fight against polarized thinking, they reduce Marcuse's complex philosophy to a simple call to censor the Right: "The left referred to students, intellectuals, and minorities of all kinds. For Marcuse, there was no moral equivalence between the two sides. In his view, the right pushed for war; the left stood for peace; the right was the party of 'hate,' the left the party of 'humanity'" (65). This critique of Marcuse is now a standard conspiracy theory of the Right, which believes that all of our major social institutions have been taken over by a secret plot to end capitalism by spreading Marxism, and the place where this hidden revolution starts is in higher education.[33]

Thus, the so-called advocates for free speech and the diversity of viewpoints use polarizing rhetoric to support the ability of illiberal groups to circulate hate speech: "They [Leftist students] would include the withdrawal of toleration of speech and assembly from groups and movements which promote aggressive policies, armament, chauvinism, discrimination on the grounds of race and religion, or which oppose the extension of public services, social security, medical care, etc." (66). In other words, the protection of academic freedom is now considered a necessary tool for the Right to voice their discrimination and rejection of the welfare state.[34]

This defense of Right-wing rhetoric is coupled with a criticism of what they consider to be Left-wing intersectionality: "Our purpose here is not to critique the theory itself; it is, rather, to explore the effects that certain interpretations of intersectionality may now be having on college campuses. The human mind is prepared for tribalism, and these interpretations of intersectionality have the potential to turn tribalism way up" (67). While it is apparently fine to have the Right express their extreme ideology, Lukianoff and Haidt reject the theory of intersectional identity because it enhances what they call tribal thinking.[35] Although I am also critical of Left-wing ideological conformity, it is vital to treat conservative and Right-wing ideologies in the same manner.

Even if we do find the constant criticisms of white males to be a form of essentialized reversed racism, we have to realize that this rejection of Left-wing ideology does not mean that we should accept Right-wing hate speech and discrimination.[36] However, in Lukianoff's and Haidt's polarized and emotional rhetoric, the focus is often placed on extreme examples of Left-wing discourse, while conservatives and the Right are usually given a free pass. What is missing from their analysis is the fact that the reason why Republicans love to attack trigger warnings, cancel culture, microaggressions, identity politics, and political correctness is that they want to attack Democrats for censoring the speech of conservatives and people on the Right:

The combination of common-enemy identity politics and microaggression training creates an environment highly conducive to the development of a "call-out culture," in which students gain prestige for identifying small offenses committed by members of their community, and then publicly "calling out" the offenders. One gets no points, no credit, for speaking privately and gently with an offender – in fact, that could be interpreted as colluding with the enemy.

(71)

From the perspective of the libertarian Right, the Left now embodies the super-ego censoring our thoughts and words by making us feel ashamed of our aggressive impulses.[37] Although it is true that some on the Left do participate in this type of censorship and shaming, what is concerning about Lukianoff's and Haidt's approach is that it claims to be defending everyone's free speech when, in reality, it is mostly concerned about having conservatives and Right-wingers play a larger role in higher education.[38] If they were really advocates of universities and academic freedom, they would argue that no ideology should be used to guide the pursuit of truth through reason except the anti-ideology ideology of modern science.[39]

In terms of the college mental health crisis, Lukianoff and Haidt are not only arguing that students are being coddled by protective administrators, but they also feel that these administrators are driven by a narcissistic mode of virtue signaling:

> We can begin to see the way that social media amplifies the cruelty and "virtue signaling" that are recurrent features of call-out culture. (Virtue signaling refers to the things people say and do to advertise that they are virtuous. This helps them stay within the good graces of their team.) Mobs can rob good people of their conscience, particularly when participants wear masks (in a real mob) or are hiding behind an alias or avatar (in an online mob). Anonymity fosters dein-dividuation – the loss of an individual sense of self – which lessens self-restraint and increases one's willingness to go along with the mob.
>
> (73)

In the passage, the narcissistic desire of administrators to look good is confused with the mob mentality of activist groups that seek to produce solidarity by remov-ing reality testing and the individual's morality in favor of the group mind. As Freud insists, in extreme forms of love and group solidarity, individuals suspend their own reason in favor of an idealized Other.[40]

The Republican Attack on Unions and Minorities

While this form of extreme group tribalism can occur on the Left and the Right, Lukianoff and Haidt emphasize its role in the Democratic Party:

> Mark Lilla points out in his book he *The Once and Future Liberal: After Identity Politics*, they are not enough to bring about lasting change. You have to win elections to do that, and to win elections, you have to draw in very large num-bers of people from diverse groups. Lilla argues that the left did that success-fully from the presidency of Franklin D. Roosevelt through the Great Society era of the 1960s, but then it took a wrong turn into a new, more divisive, and less successful kind of politics: Instead they threw themselves into the movement politics of identity, losing a sense of what we share as citizens and what binds us as a nation. An image for Roosevelt liberalism and the unions that supported it was that of two hands shaking. A recurring image of identity liberalism is that of a prism refracting a single beam of light into its constituent colors, producing a rainbow. This says it all.
>
> (81)

The main argument here is that the Democratic Party has given up an older form of liberal pragmatism in favor of a Leftist mode of identity politics, and this new poli-tics is counter-productive because it relies on extreme, uncritical groupthink. How-ever, what this theory leaves out is that the Democratic Party has always combined together radicals and moderates, and what has caused the party to stop advocating for the working class in order to protect the interests of upper-middle-class professionals is the loss of unionized workers and their political contributions.[41] Moreover, what has helped to cause this loss of union power is a long effort by the Republicans to deny union rights and the ability of workers to form these collective organizations.[42] The issue, then, is not that the Democrats have become more extreme through their commitment to minority rights: The main problem is that the Republicans have become more effective at demonizing the welfare state and union protections, and both of these efforts are tied to the claim that the government is the problem and not the solution.[43]

Behind the attack on unions, the welfare state, and minority-based social movements, we find a tax revolt led by the wealthiest Americans.[44] Since these libertarians wanted to be free from taxes and regulation, they had to argue that government spending could be reduced, and this was possible because they claimed that most of the taxes are used to support welfare programs going to people of color.[45] Since they also argued that we no longer really have prejudice and discrimination, welfare aid for minorities could be eliminated. When people pointed to the continuing issue of racism, the Right simply countered that people were just being overly sensitive, and here is where the attack on microaggressions comes in.[46] Due to the fact that it is necessary for the Right to deny racism in order to defund the welfare state and reduce the taxes of the wealthy, they have to posit that any claim of racism is the product of a paranoid, super-sensitive mind – or Left-wing indoctrination.[47]

It is vital to ground our understanding of the student mental health crisis and the administrative narcissistic accommodations to this hysteria within this political culture war. While conservatives want students to toughen up and respect traditional sources of authority, Lukianoff and Haidt emphasize how Leftist politics is pushing students and faculty to censor people on the Right who are seen as being insensitive to their claims of prejudice and symbolic violence. Meanwhile, faculty who feel that all students are victims of trauma argue that we should find ways to affirm and accommodate student suffering. Student mental health has been, therefore, highly politicized and is being used by different ideologies to make very different claims.[48]

As Lukianoff and Haidt demonstrate, one of the causes for this culture war surrounding trauma and censorship deals with the notion of symbolic violence. In their analysis of a student essay on this topic, they quote the following argument: "But if asking for peaceful dialogue is violent, then it seems that the word 'violence' is taking on new meanings for some students" (85). Just as the definition of trauma has been expanded, the meaning of violence has migrated from purely physical to mostly psychological: People increasingly do not distinguish between physical acts and words, and so more individuals can claim that they are traumatized victims of violence.[49] This confusion of real and imagined violence can be explained by Freud's important theory of the primary processes because what he discovered was that on the level of thought and emotion, there is no clear distinction between representations and reality.[50] Since humans have the ability to imagine things that do not exist, they are prone to project their thoughts onto the world as they deny the fundamental goal of reason, which is to distinguish fact from fiction.

Due to the repression of psychoanalysis, this conception of thought and emotion is not understood, and so there is a lack of comprehension concerning the ways individuals and groups become irrational. Furthermore, Freud claimed that the primary processes are often unconscious, and they are not controlled by the intentional ego; in other words, people are not always masters of their own minds, and they have to learn how to become more rational.[51] The question, then, is how does a society replace irrational thinking with reason? There are two main responses to this question. The first concerns the creation of social institutions and practices dedicated to the ideals of impartiality and empiricism.[52] Thus, we want our judges and scientists to examine evidence from a neutral perspective. Likewise, it is necessary for journalists to objectively report the truth of reality and for educators to communicate knowledge and teach students how to discover the truth in an unbiased way. Of course, it is impossible to be entirely neutral, but these are the ideals of modern liberal democracy and science.

If we have social institutions and social practices dedicated to reason and the reality principle, then we do not have to rely on individual thoughts and feelings, but it is still necessary to teach these guiding principles and to make sure that they are protected. Yet, the question remains concerning how individuals can become more rational. Freud's central claim is that the only way that the reality principle can replace the pleasure principle and the primary processes is if people freely learn on their own about their unconscious minds and the fact that they are not in control of their own thoughts and emotions.[53] It is also necessary to learn how to free oneself from group thought and the idealization of leaders and ideals that prevent reality testing. In comparing the analysis to the process of mourning, Freud insisted that it is necessary to separate our distorted memories from the real world as we stop protecting idealized others or blaming ourselves for things we cannot control.

Is CBT the Solution?

Instead of affirming Freud's defense of reason, Lukianoff and Haidt turn to CBT in order to posit a way to help people to eliminate their faulty and harmful thoughts and feelings. Drawing from the work of Aaron Beck, they promote an anti-psychoanalytic model of therapy that employs the authority of the therapist to suggest different thoughts and feelings:

> He noticed that his patients tended to get themselves caught in a feedback loop in which irrational negative beliefs caused powerful negative feelings, which in turn seemed to drive patients' reasoning, motivating them to find evidence to support their negative beliefs. Beck noticed a common pattern of beliefs, which he called the "cognitive triad" of depression: "I'm no good," "My world is bleak," and "My future is hopeless."
>
> (36)

The basic idea behind this mode of therapy is to simply tell patients to change their thoughts and feelings in order to become more effective and happy.[54] This technique is then very similar to Freud's initial mode of analysis, where he would suggest to hypnotized patients what they should think and feel, but Freud realized that this coercive, superficial method did not have lasting effects because it did not deal with the underlying unconscious causes.[55]

For Lukianoff and Haidt, Freud needs to be forgotten because there is no reason to dwell on memories of the past: "At the time, Freudian ideas dominated psychiatry. Clinicians assumed that depression and the distorted thinking it produces were just the surface manifestation of deeper problems, usually stretching back to unresolved childhood conflict. To treat depression, you had to fix the underlying problem, and that could take many years of therapy" (36). Instead of examining the roots of mental issues, Beck and the practitioners of CBT believe that it is more efficient and effective for the therapist simply to tell the patient to change their current thoughts.[56] Thus, just like the conservatives and Right-wingers who think that students and minorities need to just stop having negative emotions and thoughts, Lukianoff and Haidt promote a mode of therapy that is fundamentally a form of social mind-control.[57]

Although it may appear that Beck discovered a way to make people more rational, what he did was to force them to repress their negative thoughts and feelings by replacing them with positive ideas dedicated to fitting in better with society: "Beck's great discovery was that it is possible to break the disempowering feedback cycle between negative beliefs and negative emotions. If you can get people to examine these beliefs and consider counterevidence, it gives them at least some moments of relief from negative emotions, and if you release them from negative emotions, they become more open to questioning their negative beliefs" (37). The first problem with this method is that it places the patient in the position of being dependent on an idealized authority as it gets people simply to hide their own negative thoughts from themselves and others.[58] Moreover, as Freud discovered, people do not really change if they think that the transformation is coming from someone else.[59]

Beck's model also suffers from the fact that it misunderstands the unconscious and the primary processes as it tries to train people simply to make a conscious decision to have positive thoughts and feelings: "it is possible to train people to learn Beck's method so they can question their automatic thoughts on their own, every day. With repetition, over a period of weeks or months, people can change their schemas and create different, more helpful habitual beliefs (such as 'I can handle most challenges' or 'I have friends I can trust'). With CBT, there is no need to spend years talking about one's childhood" (37). As I will discuss in the next chapter, there is a lot of evidence that this type of mind training does not work in the long term, but what I want to focus on now is how CBT dovetails with conservative and Right-wing politics.[60]

Since the goal of conservative ideology is to maintain a social hierarchy privileging white Christian heterosexual males, there is a desire to silence the complaints of women, people of color, and the LGBTQ+ community. As a defense of white patriarchy, it is necessary to censor and discipline people who have issues with the dominant cultural ideology.[61] Likewise, the libertarian Right needs to attack people pushing for diversity, equity, and inclusion because these Leftist values can threaten white male privilege as they force these individuals to care about the plight of minoritized subjects.[62] By equating the protests of minority groups with the complaints of students suffering from anxiety and depression, Republicans can gain political power as they rally around a shared hatred for what is perceived to be a Left-wing conspiracy.[63] Although they may argue that they just want to protect universities by promoting academic freedom, what they really want to do is demonize one of the only institutions that they have failed to control.[64] On a very basic level, they want to perform CBT on the students, faculty, and administrators by convincing them to replace their negative thoughts and feelings with positive ones as they learn how to conform to conservative social norms and capitalist efficiency.[65]

Lukianoff and Haidt might respond to this criticism by insisting that they are just trying to reduce polarization and irrational groupthink by teaching people how to think more rationally, but their insistence on CBT as the solution tells another story. Since they focus on how the Left and liberals use emotional reasoning, catastrophizing, overgeneralizing, and dichotomous thinking to gain group solidarity and to define a common enemy, their main targets of distorted thinking are Democrats: "Everyone engages in these distortions from time to time, so CBT is useful for everyone. Wouldn't our relationships be better if we all did a little less blaming and dichotomous thinking, and recognized that we usually share responsibility for conflicts? Wouldn't our political debates be more productive if we all did less overgeneralizing and labeling, both of which make it harder to compromise?" (39). Of course, all of the major political ideologies engage in these types of distorted thinking, but what Lukianoff and Haidt see as dominating the universities is the combination of centrist liberals and Leftist activists. The goal then is to silence these protesters and complainers by getting them to replace their negative feelings with positive ideas.

As a way of arguing against safe spaces, trigger warnings, cancel culture, microaggressions, and trauma-informed pedagogy, they argue for a university that would no longer coddle and protect students from being exposed to different ideologies:

> Learning about cognitive distortions is especially important on a college campus. Imagine being in a seminar class in which several of the students habitually engage in emotional reasoning, overgeneralization, dichotomous thinking, and simplistic labeling. The task of the professor in this situation is to gently correct such distortions, all of which interfere with learning – both for the students engaging in the distortions and for the other students in the class. For example, if a student is offended by a passage in a novel and makes a sweeping generalization about the bad motives of authors who share the demographic characteristics of the offending author, other students might disagree but be reluctant to say so publicly.
>
> (39)

Thus, the proposed solution to the student mental health crisis and cancel culture is to motivate teachers to act like practitioners of CBT, but doesn't this just enhance the power of teachers and diminish the autonomy of students? More importantly, can you simply tell someone how to be more rational or positive?

Instead of turning teachers into CBT therapists, it would be more effective to teach the principles of modern academic discourse, which relies on impartiality, empiricism, and equal treatment of every student. If we want to protect liberal democracy and science, then we have to insist on creating a space where the ideals of reason and reality testing are privileged.[66] At times, Lukianoff and Haidt appear to endorse this type of education: "There is no universally accepted definition of 'critical thinking,' but most treatments of the concept include a commitment to connect one's claims to reliable evidence in a proper way – which is the basis of scholarship and is also the essence of CBT" (39). The problem with this equating of critical thinking with CBT is that CBT tends to negate the reality of thoughts, feelings, and memories; thus, CBT simply tries to hide the truth of students' own interiority and past by replacing their subjectivity with the dictates of an authority figure. What we need to do is stop seeing education as therapy, especially when the modes of therapy being promoted repress psychoanalysis.

Notes

1 Lukianoff, Greg, and Jonathan Haidt. *The Coddling of the American Mind: How Good Intentions and Bad Ideas Are Setting Up a Generation for Failure*. Penguin, 2019.
2 Welbaum, Samuel. "The coddling of the American mind: How good intentions and bad ideas are setting up a generation for failure." *Journal of Interdisciplinary Studies* 33.1–2 (2021): 188–191.
3 Nayak, Sameera S., et al. "Is divisive politics making Americans sick? Associations of perceived partisan polarization with physical and mental health outcomes among adults in the United States." *Social Science & Medicine* 284 (2021): 113976.
4 Biondi, Carrie-Ann. "The coddling of the American mind: How good intentions and bad ideas are setting up a generation for failure." *Reason Papers* 41.2 (2020): 76–86.
5 Nascimento, Victor. *The Hegemony of the Neoliberal Narrative: Right Wing Discourses of 'Common Sense', the Weaponization of the Term 'Liberal', and the Shifting of the Political Spectrum*. Diss., University of Victoria, 2021.
6 Pascale, Celine-Marie. "The weaponization of language: Discourses of rising right-wing authoritarianism." *Current Sociology* 67.6 (2019): 898–917.
7 Conason, Joe. *Big Lies: The Right-Wing Propaganda Machine and How It Distorts the Truth*. Macmillan, 2004.
8 Herbert, John M. "Academic free speech or right-wing grievance?" *Digital Discovery* 2.2 (2023): 260–297.
9 Samuels, Robert, and Robert Samuels. "Logos, global justice, and the reality principle." *Zizek and the Rhetorical Unconscious: Global Politics, Philosophy, and Subjectivity*. Springer, 2020, 65–86.
10 Schwartz, Victor, and Jerald Kay. "The crisis in college and university mental health." *Psychiatric Times* 26.10 (2009): 32–32.
11 Strossen, Nadine. "Resisting cancel culture: Promoting dialogue, debate, and free speech in the college classroom. Perspectives on higher education." *American Council of Trustees and Alumni*. Routledge, 2020.
12 Campbell, Bradley, and Jason Manning. "The rise of victimhood culture." *Microaggressions, Safe Spaces, and the New Culture Wars, The Rise of Victimhood Culture: Microaggressions, Safe Spaces, and the New Culture Wars* 1 (2018): 265.

13 Anderson, R. J. *Dark Psychology: Master the Advanced Secrets of Psychological Warfare, Covert Persuasion, Dark NLP, Stealth Mind Control, Dark Cognitive Behavioral Therapy, Maximum Manipulation, and Human Psychology*. Alakai Publishing LLC, 2020.
14 Freud, Sigmund. "The history of the psychoanalytic movement." *The Psychoanalytic Review (1913–1957)* 3 (1916): 406.
15 Leuzinger-Bohleber, Marianne, et al. "Outcome of psychoanalytic and cognitive-behavioural long-term therapy with chronically depressed patients: A controlled trial with preferential and randomized allocation." *The Canadian Journal of Psychiatry* 64.1 (2019): 47–58.
16 Orlenius, Kennert. "Tolerance of intolerance: Values and virtues at stake in education." *Journal of Moral Education* 37.4 (2008): 467–484.
17 Prasko, Jan, et al. "Transference and countertransference in cognitive behavioral therapy." *Biomedical Papers* 154.3 (2010): 189–197.
18 Prasko, Jan, et al. "Transference and countertransference in cognitive behavioral therapy." *Biomedical Papers* 154.3 (2010): 189–197.
19 Freud, Sigmund. *Group Psychology and the Analysis of the Ego*. WW Norton & Company, 1975.
20 O'Loughlin, Michael. *CBT: The Cognitive Behavioural Tsunami: Managerialism Politics, and the Corruptions of Science*. London and New York: Farhad Dalal Routledge, 1st ed., 2018, 197pp., $140, hardback, ISBN: 978-1-138-313064 (2021), 141–147.
21 Samuels, Robert, and Robert Samuels. "Pathos, Hysteria, and the left." *Zizek and the Rhetorical Unconscious: Global Politics, Philosophy, and Subjectivity*. Springer, 2020, 33–47.
22 Herbert, John M. "Academic free speech or right-wing grievance?." *Digital Discovery* 2.2 (2023): 260–297.
23 Norris, Pippa. "Cancel culture: Myth or reality?" *Political Studies* 71.1 (2023): 145–174.
24 Horwitz, Paul. "Universities as first amendment institutions: Some easy answers and hard questions." *UCLA Law Review* 54 (2006): 1497.
25 Bonikowski, Bart, and Yueran Zhang. "Populism as dog-whistle politics: Anti-elite discourse and sentiments toward minority groups." *Social Forces* 102.1 (2023): 180–201.
26 Sauer, Birgit. "Cultural war 2.0? The relevance of gender in the radical populist-nationalist right." *Capitalism in Transformation*. Edward Elgar Publishing, 2019, 169–182.
27 Tudor, Alyosxa, and Miriam Ticktin. "Sexuality and borders in right wing times: A conversation." *The Sexual Politics of Border Control*. Routledge, 2022, 164–183.
28 Campbell, Bradley, et al. "Microaggression and the culture of victimhood." *The Rise of Victimhood Culture: Microaggressions, Safe Spaces, and the New Culture Wars*. Springer, 2018, 1–36.
29 Hodson, Gordon. "Pushing back against the microaggression pushback in academic psychology: Reflections on a concept-creep paradox." *Perspectives on Psychological Science* 16.5 (2021): 932–955.
30 Lobban, Rosemary, et al. "Right-wing populism and safe identities." *NORMA* 15.1 (2020): 76–93.
31 Patterson, Kelly, Anna Maria Santiago, and Robert Mark Silverman. "The enduring backlash against racial justice in the United States: Mobilizing strategies for institutional change." *Journal of Community Practice* 29.4 (2021): 334–344.
32 Lukianoff, Greg, and Rikki Schlott. *The Canceling of the American Mind: Cancel Culture Undermines Trust and Threatens Us All – But There Is a Solution*. Simon and Schuster, 2023.
33 Rufo, Christopher F. "Bring on the counterrevolution; Conservatives need a national agenda that reclaims American institutions from the Left. A blueprint exists, from a surprising source." *City Journal* (2023): NA–NA.
34 Withorn, Ann. "Fulfilling fears and fantasies: The role of welfare in right-wing social thought and strategy." *Unraveling the Right* (2019): 126–147.

35 Lane, Justin E., Kevin McCaffre, and F. LeRon Shults. "The moral foundations of left-wing authoritarianism: On the character, cohesion, and clout of tribal equalitarian discourse." *Journal of Cognition and Culture* 23.1–2 (2023): 65–97.

36 Herbert, John M. "Academic free speech or right-wing grievance?" *Digital Discovery* 2.2 (2023): 260–297.

37 Samuels, Robert, and Robert Samuels. "Catharsis: The politics of enjoyment." *Zizek and the Rhetorical Unconscious: Global Politics, Philosophy, and Subjectivity*. Springer, 2020, 7–31.

38 Wilson, John K. "Myths and facts: How real is political correctness." *William Mitchell Law Review* 22 (1996): 517.

39 Pagden, Anthony. *The Enlightenment: And Why It Still Matters*. Oxford University Press, 2013.

40 Freud, Sigmund. *Group Psychology and the Analysis of the Ego*. WW Norton & Company, 1975.

41 Frank, Thomas. *Listen, Liberal: Or, What Ever Happened to the Party of the People?* Macmillan, 2016.

42 Gould, Lewis. *Grand Old Party: A History of the Republicans*. Random House, 2007.

43 Auerbach, Carl A. "Is government the problem or the solution." *San Diego Law Review* 33 (1996): 495.

44 Martin, Isaac William. *The Permanent Tax Revolt: How the Property Tax Transformed American Politics*. Stanford University Press, 2008.

45 Epstein, Richard A. "Taxation with representation: Or, the libertarian dilemma." *Canadian Journal of Law & Jurisprudence* 18.1 (2005): 7–21.

46 Lentin, Alana. "Beyond denial: 'Not racism' as racist violence." *Unsettled Voices*. Routledge, 2021, 9–23.

47 Cruz, Ted. *Unwoke: How to Defeat Cultural Marxism in America*. Simon and Schuster, 2023.

48 Quan, Wei, and Qiao Xie. "The problems of 'mental health trend' in the ideological and political management of college students under the network environment." *Journal of Environmental and Public Health* 2022 (2022).

49 Burawoy, Michael. *Symbolic Violence: Conversations with Bourdieu*. Duke University Press, 2019.

50 Samuels, Robert, and Robert Samuels. "The unconscious and the primary processes." *Freud for the Twenty-First Century: The Science of Everyday Life*. Springer, 2019, 27–42.

51 Freud, Sigmund. "Formulations regarding the two principles in mental functioning." D. Rapaport (Ed.), *Organization and Pathology of Thought. Selected Sources*. New York and London: Columbia University Press, 1951, 315–328.

52 Teorell, Jan, and Bo Rothstein. "What is quality of government: A theory of impartial institutions." *GOVERNANCE: An International Journal of Policy, Administration and Institutions* 21.2 (2008): 165–190.

53 Rieff, Philip. *Freud: The Mind of the Moralist*. University of Chicago Press, 1979.

54 Beck, Judith S., and J. H. Wright. "Cognitive therapy: Basics and beyond." *The Journal of Psychotherapy Practice and Research* 6 (1997): 71–80.

55 Freud, Sigmund. "The history of the psychoanalytic movement." *The Psychoanalytic Review (1913–1957)* 3 (1916): 406.

56 Beck, Aaron T. "Cognitive therapy, behavior therapy, psychoanalysis, and pharmacotherapy: A cognitive continuum." *Cognition and Psychotherapy*. Boston, MA: Springer US, 1985, 325–347.

57 Milburn, Milo C. "Cognitive-behavior therapy and change: Unconditional self acceptance and hypnosis in CBT." *Journal of Rational-Emotive & Cognitive-Behavior Therapy* 29 (2011): 177–191.

58 Prasko, Jan, et al. "Transference and countertransference in cognitive behavioral therapy." *Biomedical Papers* 154.3 (2010): 189–197.

59 Freud, Sigmund. "Analysis terminable and interminable." *The International Journal of Psycho-Analysis* 18 (1937): 373.
60 Feltham, Colin, and Richard House. "The politics of counselling psychology." *Counselling Psychology: A Textbook for Study and Practice*. Wiley, 2015, 330–345.
61 Rothman, Barbara Katz. "Beyond mothers and fathers: Ideology in a patriarchal society." *Mothering*. Routledge, 2016, 139–157.
62 Arndt, Christoph, and Jens Peter Frølund Thomsen. "Ethnicity coding revisited: Right-wing parties as catalysts for mobilization against immigrant welfare rights." *Scandinavian Political Studies* 42.2 (2019): 93–117.
63 Campbell, Bradley, and Jason Manning. "The rise of victimhood culture." *Microaggressions, Safe Spaces, and the New Culture Wars, The Rise of Victimhood Culture: Microaggressions, Safe Spaces, and the New Culture Wars* 1 (2018): 265.
64 Kamola, Isaac. "Dear administrators: To protect your faculty from right-wing attacks, follow the money." *Journal of Academic Freedom* 10 (2019): 1–24.
65 Parker, Ian. "6 Lacanian psychoanalysis and CBT." *EBOOK: Critically Engaging CBT* (2010): 72.
66 Samuels, Robert, and Robert Samuels. "Science and the reality principle." *Freud for the Twenty-First Century: The Science of Everyday Life*. Springer, 2019, 5–16.

Chapter 5

CBT as the False Answer to the Student Mental Health Crisis

As I have discussed in previous chapters, we are currently experiencing a major increase in reported student mental health issues on college campuses. One possible reason for this problem is that students are being over-diagnosed, and the hysterical desire to have suffering recognized by others is enabled by parents, educators, and therapists who want to feel good about themselves by catering to people who present mental health symptoms. We have also seen that an expanded notion of trauma and PTSD has produced a generation of young people who believe that they are victims of extreme external events. In response to these claims of victimization, we often encounter narcissistic individuals seeking to signal their virtue by responding to a generalized sense of trauma. Furthermore, as I outlined in the last chapter, many conservative and Right-wing activists believe that the increased vulnerability and sensitivity of young people is largely the result of a lack of authority coupled with a Left-wing focus on the suffering of minoritized students. In response to these political demonstrations of discontent, the response is often to call for tough love or some form of CBT to change these students' hearts and minds. In order to further examine these conflicting conceptions of student suffering and educational therapy, I will turn to Farhad Dalal's *CBT: The Cognitive Behavioural Tsunami.*[1]

CBT and the Repression of Psychoanalysis

Dalal's criticism of CBT begins with a description of how these therapists now approach mental suffering:

> If you go to your GP because of feeling depressed for some reason, in your ten-minute consultation your GP is almost certain to offer you anti-depressants or/and the 'one-size-fits-all' manualized treatment called CBT. The 'treatment' will try to teach you to replace your 'negative' thoughts with 'positive' ones. Your CBT therapist will have little interest in why you are depressed (perhaps you have been bereaved) because they think depression to be an illness, rather than a reasonable response to a devastating life event. According to the latest edition of the psychiatric bible, the Diagnostic and Statistical Manual V (DSM

DOI: 10.4324/9781003545668-5

V, 2013), if you are still grieving a whole two weeks after your bereavement, it is because you are suffering from a mental disorder, because you should have come to terms with your loss by then.

(1)

Thus, doctors and therapists have turned to CBT and away from psychoanalysis because they see this form of treatment to be much faster and cost-effective.[2] Moreover, governments, like the UK, are adopting this mode of therapy because, unlike psychoanalysis, it does not try to examine the causes of mental issues; instead, it treats symptoms by correcting what it determines to be counter-productive thoughts.[3] We also find universities and colleges turning to CBT because it offers what is perceived to be a cheaper way of dealing with the increased demand for mental health services.[4]

Dalal believes that the promotion of CBT can be partially blamed on the corruption of science at research universities:

In part, this has come about because in more recent times in some quarters of the academy, the notion of scientific knowledge itself has become progressively corrupted and degraded by the self-serving manoeuvres of a number of interest groups. This is somewhat ironic, because the function of the scientific attitude when it first emerged during the Enlightenment was precisely to expose the self-serving rationalizations of the then ruling elites to be fantastical fictions, not facts.

(1)

From Dalal's perspective, CBT has been legitimized by faculty who have perverse incentives to make false claims about its efficacy.[5] Since governments, students, and parents want to find a quick fix to perceived mental suffering, they have turned to CBT, which has been at times falsely represented by academic researchers seeking funding, publications, advancements, and raises.[6] In other terms, university science has been corrupted by self-interest, and this corruption has been hidden by self-serving rationalizations.

The problem, then, of college mental health is not only derived from students taking on a hysterical identity and faculty and administrators responding in a narcissistic fashion; what Dalal finds in the promotion of CBT is an undermining of reason and science within the very institutions that are supposed to be shaped by these Enlightenment ideals.[7] Dalal indicates that one reason for this privileging of a false scientific method and an ineffective model of mental health treatment is the repression of psychoanalysis. According to his analysis, the driving force behind all of these trends is Neoliberalism as an ideology centered on efficiency and the accumulation of wealth at any cost:[8]

A key doctrine of hyper-rationality is a distorted and amoral take on 'efficiency'. We can see it in play in the workings of neoliberalism. To begin with, neoliberalism uses a shallow and instrumentalist definition of efficiency having to do with profit and money, to rationalize and legitimate deregulation. It follows this up by calling on efficiency again to legitimate the austerity measures that are deemed to be necessary to repair the damage done by the deregulation in the first place.

(5)

From Dalal's perspective, a reduction in state welfare funding has created a great deal of human suffering, and in response to this public discontent, governments and universities have advocated for CBT as a fast and cost-effective way of changing people's minds and silencing their criticisms.[9]

For Dalal, what makes CBT so attractive to contemporary institutions and administrators is that it appears to be both scientific and capitalistic: "It is in the name of efficiency that bureaucracies fund CBT over and above the other forms of therapy, on the basis of the claim that CBT's efficacy has been scientifically demonstrated; it also just happens to be the case that CBT treatments are inexpensive and relatively quick to implement (that is, they are "efficient"). In sum, CBT is a managerialist creation, not the scientific one that it claims to be" (5). By combining together the opposing forces of capitalism and science, administrators are able to promote a form of therapy that is seen as being fast and cost-effective, but in order to legitimize this method of treatment, they have to rely on false claims coming from university researchers.[10] Moreover, institutions of higher education employ aspects of CBT in their Diversity, Equity, and Inclusion (DEI) training programs dedicated to quickly changing people's implicit and explicit biases.[11]

As Dalal demonstrates, CBT is seen as an effective solution to mental health issues and social discontent because it offers a simplified understanding of how the mind works and how to fix thoughts and feelings when they do not comply with social norms:

This is where CBT will come to the rescue: it will explain to you how your inner life works; it will then train you in techniques to control its workings. If, after all this, you still cannot control your inner life despite having understood the mechanism, then either this is of your choosing, or it is because you are still in the grip of your mental illness. In which case you will be the beneficiary of an additional diagnosis granted by the researchers: "CBT resistant."

(6)

As a way of replacing socially unproductive thoughts and feelings with productive ones, the goal of CBT is to use the authority of the therapist to motivate people to adapt to society in a more effective manner.[12] Like previous modes of behaviorism, one of the tricks employed in this process is simply to erase human subjectivity and the role that past experiences play in present psychopathologies.[13] In short, CBT is the opposite of psychoanalysis because it rejects the analytic notion that our current thoughts and feelings are shaped by unconscious memories, fears, desires, and defense mechanisms.

While Dalal believes that CBT can still be helpful for some people dealing with specific phobias, he worries that the benefits of this treatment have been greatly exaggerated:

> CBT is not entirely without virtue, and in a sense the problem is not with CBT itself, but the hype that surrounds it and the use it is put to further specific ideological, professional and political agendas. In its original avatar, the scope of CBT was limited. Its technology was developed to help people recover from phobias, such as fear of flying, obsessive behaviours, and so forth. In this it succeeds very well, and in these areas it is very often the 'treatment of choice'. Problems became apparent when CBT's ambitions expanded to colonize all forms of psychological suffering.
>
> (6)

Although I would dispute this claim that CBT is an effective short-term treatment for phobias and obsessive behaviors, what is clear is that the promotion of this form of therapy is derived from hidden ideological, professional, and political agendas.[14] In other terms, the forces behind the celebration of CBT are themselves repressed as false rationalizations are employed to cover non-scientific factors.

One reason why this mode of treatment is favored by the managerial class is that it is easy to instrumentalize in a standardized form that appears to save money and time:

> The treatment is manualized in order that it replicates the successes of treatment that was researched. Once a treatment is validated in this way, the job of delivering it to those troubled with a mental illness, is passed onto the statutory agency Increasing Access to Psychological Therapies (IAPT). IAPT also produces empirical evidence about its functioning and delivery of the treatment. It produces prodigious amounts of data that appears to demonstrate that the providers are delivering outcomes at the level that the research says should be the case.
>
> (7)

In discussing how and why the British government started to fund CBT as the treatment of choice for mental health issues, Dalal reveals the ways the privileging of this mode of therapy feeds into a managerial desire for simplicity, numerical calculations, efficiency, and cost-savings, and we find a similar trend in college mental health policies and practices.[15]

The Science of Happiness

One of the most important sources for the development of CBT is the science of happiness, which represents a move away from theories like psychoanalysis, which focus on mental displeasure and not the successful adaptation to cultural representations of contentment: "there was now a Science of Happiness which had not only discovered what made people happy, it could also teach unhappy persons the skills which would make them happy. What's not to like about a science that advocates that one's happiness is at least, if not more, important than money?" (13). In what is often called positive psychology, the new emphasis is on how to convince people to replace their negative thoughts and feelings with positive ones.[16] As we shall see, this form of mind training relies on the individual in treatment to regress to the position of the helpless child in front of the all-powerful parent. In other words, it relies on the type of idealization that Freud located in hypnosis, love, armies, churches, and political rallies.[17] Therefore, instead of following the psychoanalytic notion that analysis has to work to suspend transference and dependency, the goal of CBT is to use transference in order to suggest to the patient how to turn negative thoughts into positive ones.[18] Thus, it does not matter if one is in a dangerous situation or suffers from past bad experiences, the aim is to transform pain into pleasure.

To accomplish this goal of changing a person's thinking, the first step is to remove thoughts and feelings from contexts: "This is our first glimpse into the mechanistic mind-set that is CBT. Actions are stripped out of their contexts, contexts which make actions meaningful. Stripped of meaning, actions become empty instrumentalized techniques, so-called 'skills'" (14). As a form of behavior modification, which was first used on animals, CBT relies on removing subjectivity from human actions.[19] Once context and meaning are repressed, it then becomes easier to train people through some form of reward or punishment. In this way, the therapist can influence the mind of the patient by removing any subjectivity from the relationship. If this sounds like the way cults and authoritarian politics work, it is because these forms of social control rely on forcing people to regress to the position of being a helpless infant who is unable to use reason and test reality.[20]

As Dalal insists, behaviorism relies on treating people as instruments to be manipulated to achieve a particular outcome: "When a hug is reduced to technique to make myself feel happier, then the role of other person is rendered functional rather than meaningful: they are simply an object to be used in the service of adjusting my emotional state" (14). This mode of instrumentalized human relations turns therapy into a mode of mind manipulation where individuals are treated as objects to manipulate through punishment or reward.[21] As Lacan insists, this combination of hypnosis and instrumentalization represents the essence of fascism since leaders are taking advantage of the idealizing transferences as they treat humans as just objects to manipulate.[22] Furthermore, Lacan implies that a key to perversion is this transformation of subjects into objects, and we find this same issue in Marx's theory of how capitalism turns every relationship into one based on the exchange value.[23] As a form of dehumanization and alienation, pure Neoliberal capitalism transforms social relationships into a form of objectification and instrumental manipulation.[24]

To define the foundation of the new science of happiness and its relationship to CBT and Neoliberal ideology, Dalal turns to the work of Martin Seligman, who at one time was the president of the American Psychological Association[25]:

Seligman started his career in psychology by torturing dogs to the point of what he called "learnt helplessness" (Seligman, 1972). He did this by giving them electric shocks at random through the floor so that they were unable to escape the shocks by jumping away. This was done repeatedly until the dogs resigned all hope and lay down on the floor even whilst being shocked, simply whining. His great finding was this: that when these dogs were put in new situations where there was the possibility of escaping from the shocks, they did not try to do so. They had truly given up. The dogs were now deemed to have learnt helplessness.

(14)

In seeing humans as animals that could be trained to be helpless through the use of rewards and punishments, Seligman promoted a form of therapy dedicated to manipulating people into changing their thoughts and feelings.[26] On a certain level, we can see how capitalism also uses rewards and punishments in a similar manner as it pays people for conforming to a social order based on exchange value.[27]

For Seligman, depression is equated with learned helplessness, and so the solution to this mental issue is to train people how to be happy:

Seligman supposed that there was a corollary between learnt helplessness and depression. He thought that depression was a form of learnt helplessness due to having lived through previous experiences of helplessness. Depression was now being defined as being stuck in a state of imagined helplessness despite a change of circumstances. Depression then becomes construed of as the opposite of happiness.

(14)

While Freud did not equate depression with helplessness, he did argue that the original cause of anxiety and repression is derived from the encounter with a helpless subject in front of a real danger.[28] In fact, Freud posited that each step of development revolves around the threat of castration, but this threat is symbolic and not tied to an actual violent act of cutting off a body part. Instead, castration represents a displaced sense of being helpless in the face of some external danger.[29] Ultimately, Freud saw that castration, real dangers, and the fear of losing parental love and protection all produce anxiety, which then is repressed.[30] In contrast, depression is based on a withdrawal of interest in the world and an internalization of social morality. Moreover, he argued that melancholia is triggered when, in the act of idealizing another person, one attacks the self instead of the other.[31] Of course, all of these complicated substitutions, displacements, and reversals are lost in a theory that represses the primary processes by focusing on present thoughts, feelings, and symptoms.

CBT as a Fake Science

As Dalal explains, this repression of psychoanalysis by positive psychology and CBT has been supported by a turn to the new brain sciences:

In case you were wondering quite what happiness is, he tells us: "Happiness is feeling good, and misery is feeling bad . . . that feeling can now be measured by asking people or by monitoring their brains" (Layard, 2005, p. 6). These over-simplifications contain not only half-truths but also outright falsehoods. It is in this way that CBT manufactures and sustains its mythology. For one thing, it is quite untrue to say that the levels of activity in the brain "can be measured in standard scientific ways" which give us "precise answers". All we can do is to notice a correlation between an experience and electrical activity in a particular part of the brain. Correlation is not measurement. Nor is it particularly surprising to discover that there are neurological and physiological correlates to one's emotional and mental life. Humans are bodies after all, and brains are a part of the body. What would be mysterious is if no cerebral activity were visible in tandem with lived experience.

(22)

In confusing correlation with causation, neuroscience and evolutionary psychology often pretend to be scientific when, in fact, they rely on a rhetorical use of the primary processes.[32] As Freud discovered in his research on dreams, humans have the automatic mental ability to use association, substitution, and displacement to shape how they see themselves and the world around them.[33] The reason why dreams are so important to this theory of human consciousness is because they show that we are not fully in control of our minds, which seek out patterns and connections by using symbolic representations that are not tied directly to reality.[34] For the most part, CBT and the brain sciences repress this understanding of human consciousness and perception when they return to a biological or instrumental account of human thought.[35]

Thus, part of the repression of psychoanalysis and the promotion of CBT relies on a simplified, mechanical comprehension of the human mind: "There is no place for ambiguity and ambivalence in CBT psychology; it is linear and one dimensional; it has no patience with complexity" (23). Since people are seduced by simplified models that remove complexity, ambiguity, and ambivalence, they tend to accept neuroscience, evolutionary psychology, and CBT.[36] People also want to see themselves as good, competent, and happy, so they are prone to submit to others who offer a quick solution to their problems: "These skills consist of techniques which train us to 'directly address our bad feelings and replace them by positive feelings, building on the positive force that is in each of us, our better self'" (23). The fastest and cheapest way to transform negative thoughts into positive ones is simply to submit to the suggestions of the idealized authority, and yet this structure is also at the foundation of cults and other authoritarian group formations, and of course, the reliance on external authorities represents the opposite of modern science and academic principles.[37]

In referring to the work of the British economist and promoter of behaviorism, Richard Layard, Dalal demonstrates how positive psychology and CBT rely on a false sense of modern reason:

The treatment draws on the command and control ethos of hyper-rationality, so that the treatment is also devoid of complexity. "Human beings have largely conquered nature, but they have still to conquer themselves" (Layard, 2005, p. 9). Layard continues "The inner life ... determine[s] how we react to life ... So how can we gain control over our inner life?" (Layard, 2005, p. 184). The answer is CBT which we can use to "train ourselves in the skills of being happy" (Layard, 2005, p. 189). These skills consist of techniques which train us to "directly address our bad feelings and replace them by positive feelings, building on the positive force that is in each of us, our better self" (Layard, 2005, p. 188).

(23)

While Dalal labels Layard's technique as an ethos of hyper-rationality, it is vital to see how modern reason is defined by the ability to distinguish fact from fiction, and this notion of rationality is supposed to free individuals from their blind submission to authorities and biased ideologies.[38] Since CBT is based on subjects submitting to the suggestions of the therapist, it does not cater to reason or freedom; instead, it helps to turn people into instruments that can be controlled by people with power and authority.[39]

As Dalal indicates, one of the key ways that Layard was able to instrumentalize CBT was by translating human feelings into numbers that could be calculated and compared:

There is another point here which is easy enough to miss when Layard says "feeling can be measured by asking people". No doubt you have been doing this your whole lives; asking people: "How are you?". But Layard's kind of asking is scientific – unlike yours. But if you were to ask, "how depressed are you on a scale of one to five", then that is scientific, because the answer is a number. By this subterfuge a subjective experience is given the gloss of objectivity.

(23)

This transformation of emotions into numbers represents an important aspect of our current Neoliberal age since people are constantly asked to translate their thoughts, feelings, and suffering into specific numerical values – as if this magical transformation was objective and scientific.[40] Not only do doctors ask patients to rate their level of pain on a scale from one to ten, but universities ask their students to rate the effectiveness of teachers on a numerical scale.[41] The first problem with this type of calculation is that it is largely arbitrary, and the second issue is that it relies on accurate self-reporting, which represses the ways people lie to others and themselves.[42]

Dalal posits that contemporary psychology, especially the type taught at universities, often relies on pretending that the transformation of human experience into a specific number represents a mode of objective science:[43]

Psychology however, is untroubled by these complexities, as it takes up a simplistic version of operationalism in order to make itself seem more scientific. Intangibles of the inner life (emotions, aspirations, satisfaction, etc.) are operationalized, that is "measured" by the tangible. Mostly what these measurements consist of are questionnaires consisting of questions requiring a numerical answer. These numbers get added up to give a "score", which counts as measurement. The questionnaires themselves are referred to as "instruments", by which device they are given the semblance of scientific sounding credibility. This kind of practice is become so integral to the study of academic psychology today, that it is almost impossible to question its validity.

(24)

People, then, buy into the promises of CBT because they can be shown numbers proving its effectiveness, but much of this supposed evidence is either false or misleading.[44] In a self-fulfilling feedback loop, therapists ask people to rate their feelings constantly, and then they report any positive change in the numerical ratings as proof that a person is getting better.

This instrumentalization of human subjectivity is predicated on making the magical leap from the mental to the numerical as a false form of science is legitimated:

> Green, a critic of operationalism in psychology, points out that one of the initial intentions of operationalism was to do away with subjectivity by only attending to the objective measurable. But what psychology has done has been to turn operationalism on its head and "Instead of replacing "metaphysical" terms such as "desire" and "purpose" [they] used it to legitimize them by giving them operational definitions" (Green 2001, p. 49).

(24)

CBT, neuroscience, and evolutionary psychology have become so popular in part because they match the social desire to translate subjective experiences into specific numbers, which, in turn, allow for the capitalist exchange value to be mastered by managerial authorities.[45]

The Social Foundation of Subjective Unhappiness

One of the major problems with the theory of CBT is that it has no clear comprehension of what causes human suffering: "CBT is confused as to whether unhappiness is in itself an illness, or whether it is a symptom of an illness. Sometimes it is one, sometimes it is the other, and sometimes it seems that people are unhappy for an entirely different reason: our "habit" of comparing ourselves with others – social comparison" (25). Since CBT uses a simplified model of the human mind, it is unable to define the key terms it employs. Like the DSM manual for psychological diagnosis, the focus on symptoms represses the causes and underlying structures shaping psychopathology.[46] Furthermore, as Dalal highlights, CBT also represses social factors that may be causing individuals to be unhappy:

> There have been numerous epidemiological studies, one of the more recent being *The Spirit Level* (Pickett and Wilkinson, 2010), which show that the more unequal a society is, the more unhappy it is in the sense that it is prone to a whole range of

social ills, from teenage pregnancies, psychological and physical health problems, increase in prison populations, street violence, and so forth. One would think that the obvious solution would be to reduce the social and economic disparities between the rich and poor. Layard and Clark's "solution" avoids troubling itself with inequality or redistribution. Instead of addressing the causes of inequality, their solution is to change the thoughts of individuals, so that they are no longer troubled by the conditions they live in. We can see why their thesis is so appealing to the neoliberal elite. "If happiness depends on the gap between your perceived reality and your prior aspiration, cognitive therapy deals mainly with the perception of reality" (Layard, 2005, p. 197; italics added).

(25)

One of the dangers of CBT is that in the rush to make people feel better about their lives, real social issues are ignored, and destructive relationships are maintained.[47]

In fact, Dalal Layard quotes Layard as completely denying that social inequality can have any effect on a person's mental health: "There is as yet no clear evidence to show that inequality as such affects the happiness of individuals in a community" (26). Since Layard and other practitioners of CBT believe that happiness is only a state of mind, the solution to all problems is to be trained to repress any negative thoughts or feelings.[48] Yet, we know from psychoanalysis that repressed ideas have a tendency to return, and so each time one simply replaces negative thoughts and feelings with positive ones, there is a good chance that this negative content will return.[49] Moreover, Freud also found that it is quite draining to be on guard constantly against negative ideation.[50]

Dalal argues that CBT is essentially a way to force people to conform to the expectations of society – even when those expectations are destructive: "There is a further psycho-social predicament that humans suffer from which adds to their unhappiness – adaptation. Our happiness and pleasure in new goods – say a new car or computer – quickly palls and apparently, we revert back to our natural (measurable of course), set point of happiness" (26). In this version of the pleasure principle, we are told that once people have attained the objects of their desire, they return to their original level of satisfaction; however, what is missing from this theory is the Lacanian idea that desire can never be satisfied because it is based on an unconditional sense of lack and loss.[51] Since every object that causes our desire is predicated on an original object, which never really existed in the first place, we can never fully satisfy our wishes.

Lacan added that American psychoanalysis after World War II was reshaped by immigrant analysts who sought to assimilate into American culture, which Lacan argued was shaped by an ideology of happiness and conformity.[52] He then added that within the obsessional narcissistic structure, the underlying desire for recognition, love, and knowledge could never be satisfied since it was an unconditional demand for the other to submit to the will of the subject completely. Furthermore, the desire to conform and adapt to the surrounding social order was a recipe for alienation, envy, and frustration.[53] Of course, CBT neglects all of these dynamics because it is often centered on changing thoughts and feelings in the here and now without dealing with the past or deeper causes of mental issues.

Dalal adds that when theorists of CBT are asked to provide a deeper reason for people's negative thoughts and feelings, they often respond by turning to biology: "The other reason proposed for unhappiness is biology: the reason you are unhappy is because of your genetic makeup. Here too material social conditions are kept well out of the picture. In brief: It's your genes that give you the blues" (27). With the elimination of psychoanalysis as a possible treatment or explanatory theory, the option is often to turn to mind-control or medication since the cause for the problem is not society or individual choices:

> CBT goes out of its way to say over and over again that life experience has little to do with human suffering. "Under the influence of Sigmund Freud, many people used to think that the first six years of life were critical for our happiness in life, and that little else mattered . . . [it turns out that] Upbringing still matters, though less than was once thought" (Layard, 2005, p. 59). And apparently "As adoptees progress through life, the effect of their adoptive parents fades and the effect of their genes increases" (Layard, 2005, p. 59).
>
> (27)

By excluding life experiences and psychoanalysis, behaviorists are able to concentrate on changing immediate thoughts from bad to good.

CBT and the New Brian Sciences

Layard's combination of CBT and evolutionary psychology leads him to exclude all social and subjective factors:

> Layard cites studies that claim to show that one's capacity for happiness is pegged at a certain level by nature – that is, one's genes – and that level remains broadly stable despite the ups and downs of life, income and health. "Since the 1960s it has become increasingly clear that genes play a significant role in all mental illnesses" (Layard and Clark, 2014, p. 92). Hand over fist, mistruth follows exaggeration. "We are now at a stage where individual genes have been identified which can predispose to depression or bad behaviour" (Layard and Clark, 2014, p. 97).
>
> (27)

As I argued in *Psychoanalyzing the Politics of the New Brain Sciences*, theories derived from neuroscience and evolutionary psychology tend to support a Right-wing libertarian ideology because the importance of social factors and social welfare programs are denied.[54] Since, according to these theories, we are shaped by our genes, there is no real reason to think that education or social support will change things for the better. Moreover, since our genes mold our individual brains, then, the focus is placed on individual biology.[55] The major problem with this perspective is that it fails to distinguish between minds and brains, and so all mental autonomy is lost.

A related issue caused by a model of mental health controlled by biological determinism is that is rationalizes the present social hierarchy:

> If bad genes cause bad behaviour, then good genes will give you good experiences. "People with good genes also tend to get good experiences. Their parents are good at parenting. Their own niceness elicits good treatment from other people" (Layard, 2005, p. 58). Presumably the parents of children who have good genes are good at parenting because they have the good genes that they have passed onto their offspring.
>
> (27)

This type of genetic aristocracy has led to eugenics and other forms of discrimination based on faulty genetic theories: "Despite claims to truth and to scientific rigour, pretty much each and every one of these statements on genetics is false. No single gene has ever been found for depression, schizophrenia or anxiety. CBT has replaced what it has called psychoanalysis's unsubstantiated speculations about the inner psychological world, with its own substantiated speculation about the inner biological world" (27). Although I would reject Dalal's claim that psychoanalytic explanations of the mind have never been proven, what is clear is that neuroscience and evolutionary psychology often rely on questionable assumptions and manipulated research.[56]

It is vital to point out here that due to the high demand for mental health services at colleges and universities, cash-strapped schools turn to CBT and prescribed medication in order to save time and money, but these forms of therapy do not deal with the underlying issues, and problems continue to fester until they reach a breaking point.[57] Ironically, a major reason for this belief in CBT and biological determinism in higher education is that these same institutions are also producing the research supporting these flawed theories and treatments.[58] Driven by funding from pharmaceutical companies and government mental health agencies, researchers who support these types of treatments end up receiving the most amount of support and recognition, while people invested in psychoanalytic theories and therapies are mostly excluded.[59] The repression of psychoanalysis then has a profound effect on the college mental health crisis.

Turning to Meditation and Mindfulness

When universities are not advocating for CBT or pharmaceutical solutions, they often turn to Eastern spiritual practices as another form of changing people's minds: "The techniques that are taught are in fact meditative strategies drawn from ancient Eastern philosophies such as Buddhism and Hinduism. This is why in the third wave we find an abundance of terms like attachment, compassion, mindfulness, and acceptance" (37). As an alternative way of dealing with the college mental health crisis, the promotion of mindfulness and meditation often represents a repackaging of CBT[60]:

> CBT has stripped out and appropriated meditative practices from the philosophies and meaning worlds that have generated them and reduced them into sets of techniques and skills to be learnt. In effect, the philosophy and practice of Mindfulness has been colonized by the device of giving it the gloss of "Science". Knowledge and expertise no longer reside with monks and mendicants who have put in lifetimes of practice to achieve something akin to the state of Mindfulness. Now all one has to do is to take a twelve-week course to achieve the same ends.
>
> (38)

Since people tend to respect something that is given a scientific label, and universities are the place where science is often produced and communicated, higher education plays a significant role in promoting ineffective therapies and false models of the human mind.[61] Furthermore, by incorporating aspects of Eastern spiritual practices, CBT can appear to combine modern science with ancient wisdom.[62]

As Dalal indicates, CBT has its origins in behaviorism, and this theory is derived from the notion that there is no real difference between animal reflexes and human brains:

> John. B. Watson started out as an animal behaviourist. As we might expect of a behaviourist, Watson focused entirely and only on behaviour. He thought animals were mindless, machine-like entities and, therefore, the need to engage with them was deemed unnecessary. He observed responses triggered by particular stimuli from a detached position as befitted a scientist. But then when he started to study human beings, he did that too in exactly this way: "The behaviourist . . . recognizes no dividing line between man and brute. The behavior of man, with all of its refinement and complexity, forms only a part of the behaviorist's total scheme of investigation" (Watson, 1913, p. 158).
>
> (49–50)

While CBT looks like it focuses on the mind, what we often find is a model of the human animal based on automatic reflexes with no necessary mental content.[63] From this perspective, thoughts and feelings are just window-dressing that disguise biological reactions determined by evolution and encoded in genes.

The founder of behaviorism did everything he could to eliminate psychoanalytic theories since he did not think that consciousness, attention, motivation, or even sensation mattered: "Watson tells readers of his book Psychology from the Standpoint of a Behaviourist (1919), 'The reader will find no discussion of consciousness and no reference to terms such as sensation, perception, attention, will, image and the like. These terms are in good repute but I have found that I can get along without them . . . I frankly do not know what they mean'" (50). This anti-psychology

psychology forms the basis of CBT since it seeks to instrumentalize humans by removing context and content from a system based on biological reflexes.[64]

Along with Watson, B.F. Skinner enhanced the move to remove the human mind from psychology: "In the 1930s, B.F. Skinner joined Watson's attack on 'mentalism'. Mentalism, according to Skinner was the mistaken belief that a person could understand their actions through introspection. Introspection of course was at the heart of psychoanalysis. This was a key feature used to define the identity of Behaviourism: it was not-psychoanalysis, it was the antithesis of psychoanalysis" (50). In this repression of psychoanalysis, the entire function of self-awareness was negated in order to provide space for pure biological determinism.[65] Here, we find the opposite of mindfulness, because the idea is to erase the mind so that humans can become instruments of manipulation.

Since thought and consciousness are hard to document in a scientific manner, Skinner and other behaviorists thought that it was best simply to exclude the mental from consideration:

> Skinner and his kin were anti-Kantian mechanists; according to them the experience of choosing, of reasoning, of will and the like, were all illusory "[consciousness] has never been seen, touched, smelled, tasted or moved. It is a plain assumption, just as unprovable as the old concept of the soul" (Watson and McDougall, 1929, p. 15). "The behaviourist cannot find consciousness in the test-tube of his science. He finds no evidence anywhere for a stream of consciousness . . . We need nothing to explain behaviour but the ordinary laws of physics and chemistry."
>
> (50)

This scientific reduction of the human to physical and chemical laws represents a pure instrumentalization of what it means to be a person: "Human beings were simply animate machines to be studied from a detached scientific perspective, in order to learn how to control and manipulate behaviour by applying stimuli to generate required responses. Volition was an illusion. In this way the human subject became edited out of behaviourist investigations into human subjectivity" (50). There is something perverse about this vision of human beings being reduced to machines that can be manipulated: Not only is it dehumanizing, but its alienating objectification shows a total indifference to human life.[66]

In *The Psychoanalytic Understanding of Consciousness, Free Will, Language, and Reason,* I argued that the desire to see humans as either machines or animals blocks our comprehension of what makes us human.[67] In fact, what we learn from Freud is that the human ability to imagine things that do not exist makes us different from other animals as we are able to transcend our material world.[68] Freud also helps us to grasp the way our drives are different from animal instincts because the objects of our compulsions do not derive from nature or biology since they can be shaped by culture and personal preference.[69] From this perspective, we are not machines programmed by our genes, and due to the fact that we have a complex language, we are able to lie to ourselves and others, which also causes a break from reality and nature. Finally, humans have developed artificial institutions shaped by reason, and this ability to distinguish fact from fiction separates us from computers using artificial intelligence.

DSM and CBT

Instead of affirming these psychoanalytic insights, current psychology tends to return to a mechanical and animalistic comprehension of what it means to be human. For instance, Dalal reveals how Robert Spitzer sought to make sure that the Diagnostic and Statistical Manual of Mental Disorders (DSM) removed all references to psychoanalytic theory so that it could be seen as being more scientific[70]:

> Spitzer sought to improve the fortunes of psychiatry by jettisoning its affiliation to psychoanalysis as well as its focus on the internal psychological world. Spitzer was on a mission not only to follow in the footsteps of the behaviourists and cognitivists in focussing on the external and measurable, he was going to outdo them. He was going to make psychiatry a part of mainstream medicine, by turning it into an empirical evidence-based science.

(52–53)

One reason to try to make psychology more like medicine was that medical doctors get paid more and often have more social respect. Furthermore, people tend to believe in medical doctors more than therapists, and the focus on biological determinism frees individuals from blaming themselves for their discontent, as it also absolves society.[71]

Dalal highlights that CBT benefited from the updating of the DSM because the new categories of mental disorders focused on behaviors and symptoms and not underlying causes: "The DSM has crucial significance for the subject of this book because all CBT research is pinned onto one or other of the diagnostic categories found in the DSM. So if the DSM is found to be wanting, then so will the claims of CBT researchers and clinicians" (53). Although many people believe that the DSM is based on scientific evidence, Dalal found that most of the claims made by Spitzer may have been fabricated: "Spitzer claimed that drafts of the DSM were tested in field trials involving over 12,000 patients and 550 clinicians in 212 different facilities (Spitzer, 1980, p. 5). There is no evidence for this momentous claim" (53). In other words, the scientific foundation of the DSM may be a fraud based on false claims, and yet this manual shapes the way people are diagnosed and treated.[72]

At the heart of the DSM, we find the repression of psychoanalysis and the promotion of false scientific claims:

> Spitzer's strategy closely follows that of Beck and the behaviourists. No more would psychiatry attend to aetiology, questions of why things have gone wrong. Imponderables of this kind – explanations of difficulties – were portrayed as

the preoccupation of psychoanalysts. In lieu of explanation, psychiatry turned instead to description. Henceforth psychiatry would stay on the surface of things and construct its formulations only on the basis of what was visible, tangible and observable – symptoms, behaviours and traits – and in doing so, they would ensure that the psychiatric endeavour became objective. In this way, Descriptive Psychiatry was born.

(53)

The DSM, thus, represses psychoanalysis and replaces it with the description of present symptoms and behaviors disconnected from internal mental life or personal history.[73]

Interestingly, Dalal documents how the DSM-IV was produced through arguments and power plays and not on empirical research and testing:

Allen Frances (who became editor of DSM-IV) agrees that the loudest voices usually won out . . . The way it worked was that after a period of erosion, with different opinions being condensed in his [Spitzer's] mind, a list of criteria would come up . . . It would usually be some combination of the accepted wisdom of the group, as interpreted by Bob, with a little added weight to the people he respected most, and a little bit to whoever got there last . . . Spitzer seems to have made many of the final decisions with minimal consultation. (Spiegel, 2005: 59) Someone would yell out the name of a potential new mental disorder and a checklist of its overt characteristics, there'd be a cacophony of voices in assent or dissent, and if Spitzer agreed, which he almost always did, he'd hammer it out then and there on an old typewriter, and there it would be, sealed in stone. It seemed a foolproof plan. (Ronson, 2011, p. 250).

(54)

It is upsetting to think that so many people's lives have been affected by a diagnostic manual that only pretends to be scientific and that has its roots in the ability of one man to dominate others.

One of the effects of this manual is that it has become easier for lawyers to argue that their clients have been traumatized and now suffer from PTSD: "Lawyers belonging to the California Trial Lawyers Association wrote a paper "The New DSM-IV: Is It Easier to Prove Damages?" (von Tagle, 1995) in which they celebrated the fact that the DSM-IV made it easier to prove damages because of the enormous number of confusing subcategories contained within the diagnosis of Post Traumatic Stress Disorder (PTSD)" (56). The definition of mental disorders, therefore, has a tremendous social and individual effect, and in this particular case, the expansion of the definition of trauma and PTSD has been pushed by different political and economic forces.[74]

Dalal adds that PTSD started off as being tied to the perpetrators of violence but then moved to focus on the victims of extreme events:

When PTSD was first introduced into the DSM-III, those who were deemed subject to this "mental disorder" were traumatized soldiers. In other words, those who were traumatised primarily through being the perpetrators of vio-lence. But in DSM-IV, PTSD shape-shifted and its focus became centred entirely on the victims of violence (accidents, domestic and sexual abuse and so forth). While this shift is not unreasonable in itself, it did not come about because of scientific research, but rather through the advocacy of various pres-sure groups.

(57)

As we have seen, the way trauma and PTSD are now being defined has very little to do with actual science, even though science is often invoked to make it sound more valid and evidence-based.

Turning to Medication

In what I have called the Government University Medical Pharmaceutical Com-plex (GUMP), various vested interests share a set of perverse incentives that pro-mote questionable science, which often results in representing medication as the only solution to human discontentment.[75] As Dalal points out, even when studies reveal that these drugs have little if any long-term effect, they are still promoted and valorized: "There have been several meta-analyses of the data (for example, Kirsch et al., 2002, 2008), which unequivocally demonstrate that the advantage of SSRI's "over placebo is small, and possibly clinically meaningless" (Moncrieff, 2011, 177). Yet substantial scientific evidence of this kind is unable to make a dent in the prevailing belief system. Which is somewhat ironic given that the rhetoric of the psychiatric profession deifies positivist scientific evidence" (58). At the same time that these false sciences are being seen as truly scientific, psychoanalysis has been rejected because it is viewed as being unscientific, and yet many studies have shown that psychoanalysis provides better long-term results than CBT or medica-tion for most psychological disorders.[76]

One reason why people may think that psychotropic drugs are effective is that they tend to mask symptoms on a temporary basis:

At that time psychiatric drugs were thought to be similar to recreational drugs in that both produced altered states of consciousness in the mind. According to this model, psychiatric drugs might well be helpful, not because they reverse an underlying brain abnormality, but because the psychoactive state they induce may suppress or mask the manifestations of emotional or behavioural problems . . . psychiatric drugs . . . work, or appear to work, when they do, by putting people in a drug-induced state which is preferable . . . to whatever state they are in when drug-free.

(58)

Just as CBT seeks simply to change what people are feeling and thinking without dealing with the underlying causes, pharmaceutical solutions provide only a tem-porary, superficial change, which may be seen as curative.[77]

Dalal insists that this move to a medical, biological model for psychological issues is largely driven by a desire by psychiatrists to be seen as being part of the respected medical sciences: "Psychiatry was mimicking the course taken by organic medicine "in developing disease-specific models of treatment, psychiatry was following a general trend within medicine . . . [in this task] drugs are often credited with revolutionizing psychiatry by bringing it in line with [the rest of] medical science" (Moncrieff, 2011, pp. 176–7)" (58). Supporting this effort to turn therapy into a medical science is the production and promotion of neuroscience and evolutionary psychology at research universities. Since the new brain sciences tend to present a model based on biological determinism, they are often funded by pharmaceutical corporations and governmental grants.[78] In this context, an uncoordinated conspiracy is developed as drug companies and governments fund university research that legitimates biological explanations for mental health issues, which, in turn, allows psychiatrists to make more money by associating with the prestige that comes from medicine and science.[79]

A major problem with this whole complex is that it is often driven by unproven speculations:

Imipramine was first proselytized by Swiss psychiatrist Roland Kuhn who promoted the speculative view with no basis in evidence of any kind "that imipramine reverses the biochemical of physical substrate of depression" (Moncrieff, 2011, p. 181). With this unsubstantiated unscientific assertion, the idea of an antidepressant was born: a drug that allegedly targeted and treated the disease called depression (even whilst it sedated the patient).

(59)

It turns out that most psychotropic drugs claiming to be based on scientific evidence actually rely on unproven neurochemical theories: "The idea was further promoted by the dissemination of propaganda by prominent psychiatrists who went on record making entirely fictitious claims with no basis in reality – positivist or otherwise. For example, "[these drugs have] clear-cut effects on pathological states and almost no effect on normals", and "imipramine . . . is not merely sedative and symptomatic . . . but curative" (Deniker and Lemperiere, 1964, p. 230)" (59). It does not seem to matter that these drugs do not work and that they are based on false claims; what matters is that people believe they work because experts have told them they have been derived from scientific evidence.[80]

As Dalal emphasizes, what is really behind his medical model is not scientific reason but pure capitalistic greed:

This developing viewpoint suited the interests of the pharmaceutical industry for whom this became a lucrative commercial opportunity, and so it threw its weight behind the further medicalisation of human distress. Moncrieff concludes: Few people are aware that these [diagnostic] concepts have their origins, not in robust scientific research, but rather in the interests of a psychiatric profession desperate to cement its professional position, and in the marketing tactics of the pharmaceutical industry. Antidepressants have transformed a myriad of social and personal problems into a source of corporate profit and professional prestige (Moncrieff, 2011, p. 188).

(59)

Psychiatrists and pharmaceutical corporations thus have a great incentive to promote unscientific solutions that pretend to be valid and proven.[81] Not only can psychiatrists now make more money, but they can also gain increased prestige. Dalal adds that this system works because science inside and outside of universities is being funded by the pharmaceutical industry: " 'Ninety per cent of published clinical trials are sponsored by the pharmaceutical industry, [which means that they] . . . dominate this field, they set the tone, and they create the norms' (Goldacre, 2012, p. 174; italics added)" (60). Instead of science being a structure where evidence is examined in an objective way without self-interest or bias, university research is now often corrupted by the need to please outside funders in order to continue to receive new support.[82]

In examining the medicalization of human distress and the promotion of CBT, I hope that we are gaining a better understanding of the current college mental health crisis. Not only are students being over-diagnosed and over-medicated before they enroll in higher education, but when they arrive on campus, they expect to receive high levels of care. Since there is no way that these schools have the resources to accommodate all of these students, they tend to rely on quick solutions like CBT or medication. Ironically, these questionable therapies are often promoted and legitimated by university researchers who are incentivized to follow the money and prestige by advocating a biological, medical model of psychology. In turn, the focus on brains and genes represses psychoanalysis as a misguided theory of human subjectivity is applied. To further examine the effects of this rejection of Freud's thought, I want to look in the next chapter at how, within psychoanalysis itself, we are seeing a turn to biology and narcissistic accommodations.

Notes

1 Dalal, Farhad. *CBT: The Cognitive Behavioural Tsunami: Managerialism, Politics and the Corruptions of Science*. Routledge, 2018.
2 Stikkelbroek, Yvonne, et al. "Effectiveness and cost effectiveness of cognitive behavioral therapy (CBT) in clinically depressed adolescents: individual CBT versus treatment as usual (TAU)." *BMC Psychiatry* 13 (2013): 1–10.
3 Pilgrim, David. "CBT in the British NHS: Vague imposition or imposition of vagueness?" *European Journal of Psychotherapy, Counselling and Health* 11.3 (2009): 323–339.
4 Dickson, Joanne M., and Matthew J. Gullo. "The role of brief CBT in the treatment of anxiety and depression for young adults at a UK university: A pilot prospective audit study." *The Cognitive Behaviour Therapist* 8 (2015): e14.
5 Washburn, Jennifer. *University, Inc.: The Corporate Corruption of Higher Education*. Basic Books, 2008.
6 O'Loughlin, Michael. *CBT: The Cognitive Behavioural Tsunami: Managerialism Politics, and the Corruptions of Science*. London and New York: Farhad Dalal Routledge, 1st ed., 2018, 197pp., $140, hardback, ISBN: 978-1-138-313064 (2021), 141–147.

7 Kirp, David L. *Shakespeare, Einstein, and the Bottom Line: The Marketing of Higher Education*. Harvard University Press, 2003.
8 Smith, Sarah. "Neoliberalism and mental health care in Ontario: A critique of Internet-based cognitive behavioural therapy." *Canadian Journal of Disability Studies* 11.1 (2022): 1–25.
9 Rabeyron, Thomas. "From neoliberalism to the cognitive-behavioural tsunami in Great Britain." *Recherches en Psychanalyse* 28.2 (2019): 112a–134a.
10 Wampold, Bruce E., et al. "In pursuit of truth: A critical examination of meta-analyses of cognitive behavior therapy." *Psychotherapy Research* 27.1 (2017): 14–32.
11 Levinson, Margot. "Nine working with 'diversity' in CBT." *The CBT Handbook* 162 (2011).
12 Vyskocilova, Jana, et al. "Values and values work in cognitive behavioral therapy." *Activitas Nervosa Superior Rediviva* 57.1–2 (2015): 40–48.
13 Hager, Kristina M., and Nova Southeastern University. "Comparison of counseling theories: Psychoanalysis, gestalt therapy, and cognitive-behavioral therapy." *School Psychology: From Science to Practice* 2.4 (2010): 15–39.
14 Nadiga, Deepa N., Paula L. Hensley, and E. H. Uhlenhuth. "Review of the long-term effectiveness of cognitive behavioral therapy compared to medications in panic disorder." *Depression and Anxiety* 17.2 (2003): 58–64.
15 Smith, Sarah. "Neoliberalism and mental health care in Ontario: A critique of Internet-based cognitive behavioural therapy." *Canadian Journal of Disability Studies* 11.1 (2022): 1–25.
16 Boniwell, Ilona. *Positive Psychology in a Nutshell: The Science of Happiness: The Science of Happiness*. McGraw-Hill Education (UK), 2012.
17 Freud, Sigmund. *Group Psychology and the Analysis of the Ego*. WW Norton & Company, 1975.
18 Prasko, Jan, et al. "Transference and countertransference in cognitive behavioral therapy." *Biomedical Papers* 154.3 (2010): 189–197.
19 Moore, Jay. "The basic principles of behaviorism." *The Philosophical Legacy of Behaviorism*. Dordrecht: Springer Netherlands, 1999, 41–68.
20 Sponholz, Hai-Van Karin. *From the Inside Out: A Theoretical Study on Cults from a Depth Psychological Perspective*. Pacifica Graduate Institute, 2005.
21 Popović, Elizabeta. *Book Review: CBT: The Cognitive Behavioural Tsunami*, Routledge, 2020, 537–542.
22 Harari, Roberto. *Lacan's Four Fundamental Concepts of Psychoanalysis*. Other Press, LLC, 2004.
23 Lukes, Heather N. "Perversion, terminable and interminable: Foucault, Lacan, and DSM-5." *Discourse* 38.3 (2016): 327–355.
24 Shoikhedbrod, Igor. "Beyond fetishism and instrumentalism: Rethinking Marxism and law under neoliberalism." *Research Handbook on Law and Marxism*. Edward Elgar Publishing, 2021, 496–510.
25 Seligman, Martin. "Flourish: Positive psychology and positive interventions." *The Tanner Lectures on Human Values* 31.4 (2010): 1–56.
26 Seligman, Martin E. P., and Mihaly Csikszentmihalyi. *Positive Psychology: An Introduction*. Vol. 55, No. 1. American Psychological Association, 2000.
27 Rakos, Richard F. "Capitalism, socialism, and behavioral theory." *Behavior Analysis and Social Action* 6 (1988): 16–22.
28 Freud, Sigmund, James Strachey, and Alix Strachey. *Inhibitions, Symptoms and Anxiety*. New York: Norton, 1977.
29 Freud, Sigmund. "Introductory lectures on psycho-analysis." *Myths and Mythologies*. Routledge, 2016, 158–166.
30 Freud, Sigmund. *Civilization and Its Discontents*. Broadview Press, 2015.
31 Freud, Sigmund. "Mourning and melancholia." *The Standard Edition of the Complete Psychological Works of Sigmund Freud, 14.1914–1916*. Norton, 1917, 237–258.

32 Samuels, Robert. "Neuroscience and the repression of psychoanalysis." *(Mis) Understanding Freud with Lacan, Zizek, and Neuroscience*. Cham: Springer International Publishing, 2022, 29–62.

33 Freud, Sigmund. "The interpretation of dreams." *Literature and Psychoanalysis*. Columbia University Press, 1983, 29–33.

34 Samuels, Robert, and Robert Samuels. "The unconscious and the primary processes." *Freud for the Twenty-First Century: The Science of Everyday Life*. Springer, 2019, 27–42.

35 Smith, Kerri. "Neuroscience vs philosophy: Taking aim at free will." *Nature* 477.7362 (2011): 23–25.

36 Legrenzi, Paolo, and Carlo Umiltà. *Neuromania: On the Limits of Brain Science*. Oxford University Press, 2011.

37 Samuels, Robert. "Freud's contagion." *Viral Rhetoric: Psychoanalysis, Philosophy, and Politics after Covid-19*. Cham: Springer International Publishing, 2021, 61–77.

38 Pagden, Anthony. *The Enlightenment: And Why It Still Matters*. Oxford University Press, 2013.

39 Pilgrim, David. "CBT in the British NHS: Vague imposition or imposition of vagueness?" *European Journal of Psychotherapy, Counselling and Health* 11.3 (2009): 323–339.

40 Walkerdine, Valerie. "Neoliberalism." *Routledge Handbook of Psychoanalytic Political Theory*. Routledge, 2019, 380–391.

41 Williams, Wendy M., and Stephen J. Ceci. ""How'm I doing?" Problems with student ratings of instructors and courses." *Change: The Magazine of Higher Learning* 29.5 (1997): 12–23.

42 Sheridan, Zachariah, et al. "Examining well-being, anxiety, and self-deception in university students." *Cogent Psychology* 2.1 (2015): 993850.

43 LaCroix, Jessica, M., and Felicia Pratto. "Instrumentality and the denial of personhood: The social psychology of objectifying others." *Revue Internationale de Psychologie Sociale* 28.1 (2015): 183–211.

44 Shedler, Jonathan. "Where is the evidence for 'evidence-based' therapy? 1." *Outcome Research and the Future of Psychoanalysis*. Routledge, 2020, 44–56.

45 Samuels, Robert. *Psychoanalyzing the Politics of the New Brain Sciences*. Springer, 2017.

46 Lane, Christopher. *Shyness: How Normal Behavior Became a Sickness*. Yale University Press, 2008.

47 Schermuly-Haupt, Marie-Luise, Michael Linden, and A. John Rush. "Unwanted events and side effects in cognitive behavior therapy." *Cognitive Therapy and Research* 42 (2018): 219–229.

48 Shaw, Ian, and Hugh Middleton. "Sociological conceptions of happiness and its implications for psychotherapy and public policy." *Journal of Nursing & Care* 4.3 (2015).

49 Flavell, John H. "Repression and the 'return of the repressed'." *Journal of Consulting Psychology* 19.6 (1955): 441.

50 Freud, Sigmund. "Predisposition to the obsessional neurosis." *The Psychoanalytic Review (1913–1957)* 21 (1934): 347.

51 Ewens, Thomas. "Desire and the loss of object." *American Journal of Psychoanalysis* 47.4 (1987): 302.

52 Dervin, Daniel. "Where Freud was, there Lacan shall be: Lacan and the fate of transference." *American Imago* 54.4 (1997): 347–375.

53 Lacan, Jacques, Alan Sheridan, and Malcolm Bowie. "Aggressivity in psychoanalysis." *Écrits: A Selection*. Routledge, 2020, 9–32.

54 Samuels, Robert, and Robert Samuels. "The brain sciences against the welfare state." *Psychoanalyzing the Politics of the New Brain Sciences*. Springer, 2017, 85–114.

55 Lewontin, Richard C., Steven Rose, and Leon J. Kamin. *Not in Our Genes*. New York: Pantheon Books, 1984.

56 de Maat, Saskia, et al. "The current state of the empirical evidence for psychoanalysis: A meta-analytic approach." *Harvard Review of Psychiatry* 21.3 (2013): 107–137.

57   Huang, Junping, et al. "Interventions for common mental health problems among university and college students: A systematic review and meta-analysis of randomized controlled trials." *Journal of Psychiatric Research* 107 (2018): 1–10.

58   Samuels, Robert, and Robert Samuels. "Drugging discontent: Psychoanalysis, drives, and the governmental university medical pharmaceutical complex (GUMP)." *Psychoanalyzing the Politics of the New Brain Sciences.* Springer, 2017, 115–136.

59   Harrop, Chris, et al. "An independent audit of pharma influence in public mental health trusts in England." *Ethical Human Psychology and Psychiatry* 20.3 (2019): 156–168.

60   El Morr, Christo, et al. "Effectiveness of an 8-week web-based mindfulness virtual community intervention for university students on symptoms of stress, anxiety, and depression: Randomized controlled trial." *JMIR Mental Health* 7.7 (2020): e18595.

61   Rose, Steven, R. C. Lewontin, and Leon J. Kamin. "The politics of biological determinism." *Nature: The Nature of Human Nature* 2 (2005): 333.

62   Harrington, Neil, and Charles Pickles. "Mindfulness and cognitive behavioral therapy: Are they compatible concepts?" *Journal of Cognitive Psychotherapy* 23.4 (2009): 315–323.

63   Bartfeld, Rachel Ariella. "From squirrels to cognitive behavioral therapy (CBT): The modulation of the hippocampus." *The Science Journal of the Lander College of Arts and Sciences* 10.1 (2016): 4.

64   Malone, John C., and Andrés García-Penagos. "When a clear strong voice was needed: A retrospective review of Watson's (1924/1930) behaviorism." *Journal of the Experimental Analysis of Behavior* (2014): 267–287.

65   Skinner, Burrhus Frederic. "Critique of psychoanalytic concepts and theories." *The Foundations of Science and the Concepts of Psychology and Psychoanalysis* 1 (1956): 77–87.

66   Marx, Karl. "On surveillance capitalism, instrumentarian power, and social physics." *Political Theory of the Digital Age: Where Artificial Intelligence Might Take Us,* Cambridge University, 2023, 160.

67   Samuels, Robert. *The Psychoanalytic Understanding of Consciousness, Free Will, Language, and Reason: What Makes Us Human?* Routledge, 2023.

68   Samuels, Robert. "Freud's project." *(Mis) Understanding Freud with Lacan, Zizek, and Neuroscience.* Cham: Springer International Publishing, 2022, 7–28.

69   Nagera, Humberto. *Basic Psychoanalytic Concepts on the Theory of Instincts.* Routledge, 2014.

70   Guze, Samuel. "The neo-kraepelinian revolution." *The Psychopharmacologists 3.* CRC Press, 2020, 395–414.

71   Sociobiology Study Group of Science for the People. "Dialogue. The critique: Sociobiology: Another biological determinism." *BioScience* (1976): 182–186.

72   Scull, Andrew. "Rosenhan revisited: successful scientific fraud." *History of Psychiatry* 34.2 (2023): 180–195.

73   Burston, Daniel. "Psychiatry and anti-psychiatry: History, rhetoric and reality." *Eidos. A Journal for Philosophy of Culture* 2.2 (2018): 4.

74   Eagle, Gillian. "The political conundrums of post-traumatic stress disorder." *Psychopathology and Social Prejudice* (2002): 75–91.

75   Samuels, Robert, and Robert Samuels. "Drugging discontent: Psychoanalysis, drives, and the governmental university medical pharmaceutical complex (GUMP)." *Psychoanalyzing the Politics of the New Brain Sciences.* Springer, 2017, 115–136.

76   Leichsenring, Falk. "Are psychodynamic and psychoanalytic therapies effective?: A review of empirical data." *The International Journal of Psychoanalysis* 86.3 (2005): 841–868.

77   Nevins, Donald B. "Psychoanalytic perspectives on the use of medication for mental illness." *Bulletin of the Menninger Clinic* 54.3 (1990): 323.

78   Goldfried, Marvin R. "On possible consequences of National Institute of Mental Health funding for psychotherapy research and training." *Professional Psychology: Research and Practice* 47.1 (2016): 77.

79 Insel, Thomas R. "Psychiatrists' relationships with pharmaceutical companies: Part of the problem or part of the solution?" *JAMA* 303.12 (2010): 1192–1193.
80 Moncrieff, Joanna. "The myth of the antidepressant: An historical analysis." *De-Medicalizing Misery: Psychiatry, Psychology and the Human Condition.* London: Palgrave Macmillan UK, 2011, 174–188.
81 Whitaker, Robert. *Anatomy of an Epidemic: Magic Bullets, Psychiatric Drugs, and the Astonishing Rise of Mental Illness in America.* Crown, 2011.
82 Washburn, Jennifer. *University, Inc.: The Corporate Corruption of Higher Education.* Basic Books, 2008.

Chapter 6

Bad Therapy, Trauma, and Anti-Psychoanalytic Psychoanalysis

This chapter looks at how the repression of psychoanalysis inside and outside of higher education fuels the college mental health crisis. We shall see that by emphasizing trauma and misrepresenting hysteria and narcissism, a false model of therapy and mental disorder affects these schools. While the writers of the book *A New Vision of Psychoanalytic Theory, Practice and Supervision* believe that they are still doing psychoanalysis, it should be evident that their theories and practices have little to do with what Freud invented.[1] In fact, I will argue that their beliefs undermine our ability to fix the college mental health crisis because they fail to understand why and how humans use suffering to gain a sense of identity while they unconsciously manipulate others on an emotional level. Moreover, the kind of therapy they present matches many of the educational responses to trauma that we are currently encountering. In turning to Abigail Shrier's *Bad Therapy*, I will examine some of the ways the confusion of parenting with therapy has shaped contemporary college students and higher education institutions.[2]

The Talking Body

Brothers and Sletvold begin their book by positing that when psychoanalysts center their attention on bodies and body language, the meaning and goals of therapy are transformed:

> What changes when we view psychoanalytic theory from the lens of embodiment? Nothing – and everything! While there is no disputing the enduring relevance of the concepts that have become known as interpretation, dissociation, transference and resistance, we believe that they are radically transformed when a body-based approach replaces traditional concept-based theorizing. In this book we attempt to illuminate these transformations by showing how our bodies and those of our patients "talk" to one another – sometimes with words and sometimes without them – and that our conversations are always affected by the world.

(1)

DOI: 10.4324/9781003545668-6

This emphasis on how bodies communicate with each other represents a major turn away from several key concepts of psychoanalysis and relates to the recent focus on bodies, trauma, and biology in higher education.

The first way that this turn to body language moves away from classic psychoanalysis is that in Freud's final version of analytic treatment, the analyst sits behind the patient and cannot see much of the subject's body.[3] Freud first claimed that he decided to position himself in this way because he could not stand being stared at all day, but as Lacan insists, this positioning of the analyst out of the view of the patient has the benefit of making it hard for the patient to try to read the body language of the analyst.[4] As a way of breaking the imaginary mirroring between the analyst and the patient, the removal of the analyst from view places the analyst in the position of being an unknowable object, and this not only aids neutrality but also can block the narcissistic desire for recognition from the other.

As Freud discovered, without the neutrality of the analyst, there can be no free association, and without free association, it is difficult to discover what has been repressed into the unconscious.[5] Moreover, a mirroring, reflecting relationship tends to reinforce what the patient already thinks, knows, and feels by catering to an imaginary mode of empathy.[6] Since the goal of analysis is to discover something new, mirroring and restating only function to reinforce what is already known. Furthermore, when the analyst tries simply to occupy the position of the one who knows, recognizes, and cares, transference dependency is enhanced as the analyst can take on the position of the all-powerful authority in relation to the helpless subject.[7]

As I have argued in previous chapters, the repression of psychoanalysis pushes people to promote forms of therapy and education that are often counter-productive, and here we see how a turn to the new brain sciences mixed with research on infants and a misunderstanding of narcissism and hysteria can result of the destruction of psychoanalysis from within a discourse that claims to be psychoanalytic: "We believe that a 'turn' toward embodiment is gaining momentum in our field, undoubtedly spurred by the rising influence of research in neuroscience and infant development" (1). In relying on university research done on infants and brains, we run into the issue of removing talk from the talking cure. After all, as Lacan points out, "infant" means one without language, and what defines psychoanalytic treatment is that the only tool is speech.[8] The analyst then does not interpret body language, and the only way the body enters into the analysis is when it is translated into language.

One reason why these psychoanalysts want to remove speech from analysis is that they believe that a focus on trauma returns us to a type of pathology that blocks symbolization and thought.[9] In fact, the first indication of the importance of trauma to their theory and practice comes in the following statement: "Like many people in our field, I discovered that what led me to enter psychoanalytic treatment were my childhood traumas" (2). In seeing trauma as the center of analysis, they participate in the general expansion of the meaning and ubiquity of this term: "I realized that I had neglected two crucially important aspects of trauma: its intergenerational transmission as reflected in our cultural, political, historical situatedness and the fact that trauma profoundly disrupts our bodily functioning" (2–3). Not only is trauma considered to be a common cause of mental suffering and the disruption of the body, but the source of trauma has spread to intergenerational causes.[10]

By focusing on trauma, they are able to argue for a form of analysis that does not rely on speech: "I discovered that therapists and patients convey their traumatic experiences from body to body in ways that cannot be communicated verbally. Not only is it possible for therapists to gain some understanding of their patients' suffering through automatic imitation, but they communicate this understanding to their patients" (3). Instead of concentrating on the speech of the patient as the medium of analysis, the new proposed method is for the analyst to imitate what the patient's body is communicating. As we have seen, this focus on the unsymbolized body and unrepresentable trauma also structured the current trend of trauma-informed pedagogy and the general interest in trauma in the humanities.

If this method appears to be highly mystical and intuitive, it is because it relies on a magical form of bodily communication. In a mode of narcissistic mirroring, this mode of therapy imagines an empathic connection derived from imitation and intuition:[11]

Jon's writings on embodied supervision were particularly meaningful for me insofar as they demonstrated that by feeling themselves into their patients' bodies and re-experiencing their own bodily reactions in relation to them, therapists discover what had caused therapeutic impasses and misunderstandings. This approach allows therapists to become aware of how their own bodies carry traumatic meanings that may impede their work.

(3)

An essential problem with this method is that it does not allow for the neutrality of the analyst or the free association of the patient; rather, we witness a return to a magical and mystical type of communion, which is in part based on the way mothers interact with infants without speech and through mirroring.[12] In many ways, what we are witnessing here is the opposite of psychoanalysis, and yet the authors insist that they remain faithful to Freud's theories and practices.

The type of psychoanalysis that is privileged here derives in part from Kohut's notion of self-psychology, which emphasizes mirroring relationships: "In Kohut's self-psychology, I found a psychoanalytic perspective that appealed to me because, like Rogers' client-centered therapy, it focused on empathy and relationships" (4).[13] While it is true that many forms of therapy rely on empathy, psychoanalysis posits that empathy is often an imaginary projection of one's thoughts and feelings onto others.[14] Moreover, in the structure of narcissism, people seek to have their own ideal ego recognized by others by getting them merely to affirm their goodness.[15] In this relationship, the other is reduced to being an empty mirror receiving the projections of the desiring subject. In fact, one of the major revisions that Lacan made to Freud's theory of analytic treatment was to argue that the narcissist wants a neutral Other, and so it is necessary to interrupt this process by having the analyst act in some ways that breaks a sense of being dead and empty but does not feed the transference desire to embody the one who knows.[16] The trick, then, for the analyst is not to judge the patient's words while still challenging the desire to neutralize the presence of the Other.

A Return to Trauma

In their revision of psychoanalysis, the authors call for a return to Freud's original theory that all of his female patients were traumatized by being sexually assaulted by their fathers: "I argued that psychoanalysis should embrace Freud's initial trauma-based hypotheses regarding the cause of neurosis rather than his later theories about inborn conflicting drives" (4). Instead of affirming the notion that people may imagine their abuse and that neurotics suffer from conflicts between their different drives and social morality, the idea here is simply to reinforce the traumatized victim.[17] There are several problems with this approach, and one concerns the over-generalization of trauma coupled with the desire to replace all other causes of mental suffering. Although it may be easier to always side with the victim of trauma, there is still the question of how real and imagined suffering is used to justify aggression and avoid any criticism.[18] In fact, a problem with the current situation regarding sexual assault on college campuses is that we have no way of knowing how prevalent it actually is, and anyone who even suggests that some people may be imagining their abuse comes under immediate attack.[19] Part of this problem stems from the fact that most people simply do not understand the hysteria and the ways suffering can be used to gain an identity and to manipulate others in an indirect manner. While this theory can result in victim blaming, the main issue for psychoanalysis is how people respond to their real and imagined trauma.

Due to a narcissistic desire to be seen as good people, university administrators and staff tend only to affirm the trauma and responses of the people who present themselves to campus mental health providers.[20] However, instead of either affirming or denying what has happened, psychoanalysis asks us to remain neutral so that the subject can explore their thoughts and feelings in a safe space where they will be neither judged nor affirmed; of course, this neutrality does not work in a law enforcement context, and this is one reason it may be best for institutions of higher education to refer all sexual assault cases to legal authorities.[21] In terms of psychoanalytic practice, while the first response to someone presenting a trauma should be a face-to-face interview, eventually, when someone is placed on the couch, the idea is to remove the person from their normal way of communicating with friends or family members. Even though the presence of the analyst can never be completely ignored, the desire of the analyst remains unknown as the fundamental desires of the patient are allowed to emerge.[22] When the therapist simply reflects back what the patient is saying and doing, there is no space for unconscious content to surface.

Instead of asking analysts to try to occupy the position of being a non-judging presence, these authors argue that therapists should focus on their own bodily feelings and thoughts: "We then offer a new approach for describing clinical situations based on this suggested language. This involves selecting a critical moment in the therapeutic exchange and first focusing on one's own bodily reactions to a patient, then "becoming" the patient through imitation, and finally visualizing the interaction between oneself and the patient" (5). This whole process goes against most of the traditional modes of psychoanalysis since it places a lot of focus on the internal life of the analyst and an imaginary identification formed through intuition. As some critics of empathy have pointed out, when someone is thinking that they can share the same thoughts and emotions as someone else, they are often projecting their own ideas onto others.[23] This mode of narcissism functions to negate the other as the self is projected onto the neutralized Other.

My fear is that many forms of therapy and trauma-informed pedagogy are also replacing an emphasis on speech and the discovery of unconscious material with a dedication to an imaginary, narcissistic relationship.[24] According to this privileging of intuition and the body over speech, it is essential to focus on felt emotions:

> We believe that we have identified one of the main reasons that embodiment cannot be fully understood from the vantage point of existing psychoanalytic theory: traditional psychoanalytic language does not easily lend itself to embodied experience. That is, it consists of words or phrases that do not readily allow readers or speakers to feel the meaning of what is communicated in their bodies. Some common examples of concept-based language are such widely used terms as "intersubjectivity," "object relations," "the field," "the third" and "mentalization." While we recognize the need to use such words and concepts in certain contexts in order to communicate complex ideas, we believe that they sometimes obscure the human experiences they intend to explicate.
>
> (10)

Of course, all words never fully capture a real experience, but that does not mean that we should give up on speech and rely on our bodily feelings. It appears that underlying this emphasis on trauma, body language, intuition, and mirroring, we find a desire for a mystical, magical connection between people.[25]

Fixation on the Body

Not only do these authors believe that bodies can communicate in an effective manner without speech, but they also believe that language is always tied to a bodily experience:

> Our view is also highly congruent with the work of Lakoff and Johnson (1980, 1999), who developed the notion that semantics emerges from the experience of the body interacting with the environment. In their book, *Metaphors We Live By* (1980), they not only demonstrate the prevalence of metaphors in everyday language but also that our ordinary conceptual system, in terms of which we both think and act, is fundamentally metaphorical and body-based in nature.
>
> (11)

In claiming that our use of metaphor is body-based, there is an effort to once again replace the symbolic with the real and the imaginary.[26] According to this theory, language does not transcend the body or natural reality, and yet Freud's theory of the primary processes is predicated on how humans use symbolic association, substitution, and displacement to conjure a mental world that goes beyond material reality.[27]

Moreover, as Freud discovered in his work with hysterics, they often had symptoms that did not make any anatomical sense.[28] Thus, our relationship to our body is not purely natural or material, and as Lacan showed, we never really see our own body completely; instead, we rely on mirrors, pictures, and other people's perspectives.[29] As we learn from phantom limbs, our relation to our own body is based on internalized mental maps and not material reality or tested empiricism. In fact, much of Freud's work revolves around seeing the body as something mediated by culture, imagination, and desire, and so the very notion of the human body has to be seen in a complex manner.

To justify their uses of empathy and imaginary mirroring, Brothers and Sletvold return to Freud's concept of identification: "Freud was well aware of the power of imitation. He wrote: A path leads from identification by way of imitation to empathy, that is, to the comprehension of the mechanism by means of which we are enabled to take up any attitude at all towards another mental life" (12). The problem with this reference to Freud's theory of identification is that when he discusses empathy, he is highlighting a hysterical form of imitation where someone imagines that they are suffering from the same loss or emotion.[30] This type of mirroring is the opposite of analysis since nothing new is discovered as people imagine that they are sharing the same feelings.

To further rationalize their use of empathic identification, they cite the questionable theory of mirror neurons: "More recently, research on mirror neurons (Gallese, 2009) and imitation in early infancy (Meltzoff & Decity, 2003) has given strong support to the view that we learn to know both ourselves and others, both I and you, by attending to the feeling of our bodies (Sletvold, 2014, Nebbiosi & Federici, 2008)" (12–13). In this reference to the neuroscientific ideas of mirror neurons, we see how the undermining of psychoanalysis from within psychoanalysis often occurs through the use of biological determinism and unproven theories.[31] Furthermore, by focusing on the body and the infant, the understanding of emotion, empathy, and psychoanalysis are removed from symbolization and culture: "We believe our humanness is largely the result of our capacity to feel ourselves into the bodies of others, our capacity for empathy" (13). Instead of highlighting the ways humans use language and thought to shape their experiences, the desire here is to return to an imagined relationship between the infant and the empathic other.[32]

As we find in the current focus on trauma in higher education, one of the effects of this emphasis on bodies, empathy, emotion, and intuition is that reason and reality testing are suspended, and in this loss of modern rationality, a regression to magical thinking is enabled.[33] At the same time the reality principle is being repressed, there is also a negation of Freud's conception of the unconscious: "Freud's understanding of the prevalence of unconscious experience remains the cornerstone of psychoanalytic practice to this day. Wide support for the idea of unconsciousness is to be found in the work of many contemporary neuroscientists such as Damasio" (15). The problem with this reference to Damasio's understanding of the unconscious is that unlike Freud, Damasio does not equate the unconscious with repression, and like many other academic brain scientists, he uses the term unconscious to indicate brain functions of which we are not aware.[34] Of course, for Freud, the reason why we lack awareness of certain thoughts and feelings is that we are hiding them from ourselves because they threaten our self-image.[35] Most brain scientists and therapists simply repress this notion of repression because they do not want to accept the fact that a person can lie to themselves.[36]

An example of the repression of repression can be found in Bothers and Sletvold's basic theory of therapy: "Bodies do not talk to one another in the big-picture, concept-based language of psychoanalytic theory. They communicate in moment-to-moment exchanges much like those that are captured in Beatrice Beebe's descriptions of mother-infant interactions" (16). One of the things lacking in this description of analysis is the fact that people not only deceive the analyst but also deceive themselves, and so the turn to free association is supposed to create a space for people to speak without self-censorship.[37] However, if therapists focus simply on the experience of the here and now, they not only lose the connection with memories but also make it hard for people to discover their repressed thoughts and feelings. This same naïve non-psychoanalytic perspective structures many of the ways higher education thinks about students and mental health since they tend to treat expressions of present suffering and not look at the underlying structures and pathologies.[38]

In returning to the primal relation between the infant and the mother, one result is that the paternal resolution of the Oedipus complex is excluded as the emphasis is placed on the mother identifying with the child.[39] In returning to this notion of paternal intervention, it is not necessary to rely on men as the patriarchal representations of law; instead, following Lacan, we can affirm that it is necessary for someone – male or female – to transcend the mirroring relation between the child and its imaginary other.[40] This theory of the resolution of the Oedipus complex has been rejected by mostly feminist analysts and critics who want to challenge traditional gender roles, but what is often lost in this repression of the paternal role is any way to overcome the destructive aspects of empathic mirroring.[41] For example, when pedagogical theorists insist that teacher should simply affirm their students to raise their self-esteem, they often ignore the important roles that judgment and criticism play in learning.

The call for teachers to concentrate on their students' suffering often has the paradoxical effect of making the teacher focus on their own thoughts and feelings. As Bothers and Sletvold insist in relation to their vision of psychoanalysis, they recommend that instead of the analysts trying to remain neutral, they should dwell on their own thoughts and fantasies: "We try to describe what we become aware of in our bodies as well as our thoughts and fantasies in as complete a way as possible" (16). The paradox of empathy is that the more one thinks that one is thinking about the other, the more one thinks about oneself.[42] In other words, teachers, parents, and therapists who think that empathy is the solution to human suffering usually end up simply projecting their own internal experiences onto others.

Bothers and Sletvold go as far as arguing that the analyst should imitate the bodily gestures of the patient in order to share their thoughts and feelings: "Next, in "the you position," we attempt to "become" our patient by imitating the patient's facial expressions, gestures, movements and his or her way of speaking. We describe what we have experienced in our bodies as well as feelings and thoughts that occur to us as we imitate the patient" (16). This type of magical mind-reading and intuitive empathy is very different from Freud's emphasis on analytic neutrality and the free association of the patient. On a basic level, this conception of psychoanalysis represents a return to unreason and magical thinking.[43] Just as we are currently witnessing a political backlash against reason and science, we find, in this mystical retreat, a desire to return to an animistic conception of the world.[44] For higher education, this rejection of reason can only spell trouble, and yet it is often within universities and colleges that we can find the roots of this desire to be irrational.

When schools see their students as victims of some trauma, and they try to then heal the students' suffering through acts of empathy and virtue signaling, the importance of abstract thought, reason, and reality testing is repressed.[45] The same problems happen when analysts seek to return to some imagined intuitive communication between mothers and infants through bodily imitation: "Finally, in the 'we position,' we attempt to envision the exchange between ourselves and the patient by keeping in mind how we felt with the patient and how we felt when we imitated the patient" (16). In communicating their own feelings to the imitated patient, these analysts remove reason, knowledge, and reality testing from the process as they regress to an imagined state of empathic identification.[46] In this relationship, instead of the analyst remaining silent and out of view, the analyst becomes the center of attention.

In an example of how the use of empathy can be based on the narcissism of the analyst, we find Brothers relating the following: "When Amy had appeared in my office for our in-person sessions, I could not help but notice how her stylish clothes and skillfully applied makeup enhanced her striking good looks. Since I am also careful about how I dress and always wear makeup, I had assumed that we had both been subjected to similar cultural and familial pressures" (22). Instead of the psychoanalyst suspending all judgment of the patient, Brothers reveals that she was envious of her patient's looks.[47] She also admits that she assumed that because they both wanted to look a certain way, they must both share the same cultural and familial influences. The danger of judging someone based on their appearance should be obvious, but in Brothers' technique, there is a heightened emphasis on personal appearance.

One of the side effects of concentrating on personal appearance is that one can become paranoid concerning how one appears to others.[48] Brothers demonstrates this form of self-conscious anxiety in the following discussion of her case: "As I (Doris) look at Amy on the screen for the first time after the pandemic necessitated our switching to online sessions, I become aware that my smile feels forced and exaggerated.

The relaxed feeling I have had throughout my body in sessions with Amy has disappeared. I cannot find a comfortable way to sit" (22). Brothers' discomfort with her own body stems in part from her sense that her efforts to look good and smile feel forced: Her anxiety is clearly related to the anticipation of the harsh judgments of others. On one level, we can locate a narcissistic desire to have the good self recognized by the Other, but on another level, hysteria is revealed through dissatisfaction with the self, while anxiety emerges from the threat of being judged.[49]

Like so many contemporary students, especially female students, the pressure to look good for others can result in a state of constant self-scrutiny, which produces anxiety and can result in a mode of hysteria.[50] Since social media often relies on people posting images of themselves for others to like or reject, one can take on a paranoid perspective by thinking that others are always monitoring one's appearance.[51] In Brothers' case, she highlights the effects on women of the pressure to conform to cultural beauty norms: "I (Amy) turn my face to the side that makes me look more attractive in photos. I must look my best for Doris. I worry that my makeup will not disguise the asymmetry of my features. I wonder if she still likes me and wants to help me" (23). In imagining what her patient is thinking, Brothers clearly projects her own thoughts and feelings onto this other. Of course, one reason why analysts sit behind their patients is to avoid this type of narcissistic mirroring, but for Brothers, this form of imaginary identification represents the key to analytic practice.

Bad Therapy, Parenting, and University Counselling

The risk of face-to-face therapy is that it can make the patient highly self-conscious and paranoid, and it is this type of therapy that is often prevalent at university counseling centers.[52] To further examine this issue, I want to turn to Abagail Shrier's *Bad Therapy* where she outlines many of the problems with the most common therapeutic practices.[53] Shrier begins her work by calling into question the very notion that we are currently experiencing a mental health crisis in relation to young adults:

> Talk of a "youth mental health crisis" often conflates two distinct groups of young people. One suffers from profound mental illness. Disorders that, at their untreated worst, preclude productive work or stable relationships and exile the afflicted from the locus of normal life. Theirs is a crisis of neglect and undertreatment. These precious kids require medication and the care of psychiatrists. They are not the subject of this book. This book is about a second, far larger cohort: the worriers; the fearful; the lonely, lost, and sad. College coeds who can't apply for a job without three or ten calls to Mom.
>
> (xi)

The first move that she makes is to distinguish between people who need psychiatric care and others who are fearful, lonely, lost, and sad. On a most basic level, her argument is that we have broadened the definition of trauma to such an extent that we have lost the ability to separate severe mental illness from what can be considered to be "normal" mental health issues.[54]

One of Shrier's main arguments is that a social focus on the feelings of individuals often results in the production of a negative view of the self and the external world:

> When we were little, my brother and I were spanked. Our feelings were seldom consulted when consequential decisions about our lives were made – where we would attend school, whether we would show up at synagogue for major holidays, what sort of clothes fit the place and occasion. If we didn't particularly relish the food set out for dinner, no alternate menu was forthcoming. If we lacked some critical right of self-expression – some essential exploration of a repressed identity – it never occurred to either of us. It would be years before anyone in my generation would regard these perfectly average markers of an eighties childhood as vectors of emotional injury.
>
> (xv)

While Shrier's perspective can be read as a conservative defense of what is now seen as harsh parenting, her overall view helps us to comprehend how a changing conception of parenting has emphasized emotions over reason and authority.[55] Moreover, an expanded definition of "emotional injury" has paved the way for a therapeutic culture in higher education bent on seeing most students as suffering from a traumatic history.[56]

Much of her analysis relies on a generational divide, where an older model of psychology and parenting has been replaced by a turn towards therapy and feelings: "But as millions of women and men my age entered adulthood, we commenced therapy. We explored our childhoods and learned to see our parents as emotionally stunted. Emotionally stunted parents expected too much, listened too little, and failed to discover their kids' hidden pain. Emotionally stunted parents inflicted emotional injury" (xv). From this perspective, people have started to see their childhoods as inherently traumatic, and in order to reverse this suffering, they went to therapy, and parents began to think that their main role was catering to the needs and desires of their children.[57] Even though objectively, we can say that people have never lived longer lives with more rights and protections, there is a sense in the developed West that individuals are suffering mental pain at a higher rate than before.[58]

One possible explanation for this dichotomy between physical health and mental health is that once a certain level of general subsistence is met, people turn inward to examine how well they are doing.[59] Thus, in the countries where people have the longest expected lifespans, we find a high incidence of anxiety, depression, and suicide.[60] Shrier does not consider this historical factor, but she does concentrate on how our current notions of parenting may be shaped by counter-productive psychological theories:

> We never doubted that we wanted kids of our own. We vowed that our child-rearing would reflect a greater psychological awareness. We resolved to

listen better, inquire more, monitor our kids' moods, accommodate their opinions when making a family decision, and, whenever possible, anticipate our kids' distress. We would cherish our relationship with our kids. Tear down the barrier of authority past generations had erected between parent and child and instead see our children as teammates, mentees, buddies.

(xv)

Behind this drive of parents to treat their children as friends, we often can locate a narcissistic desire for adults to re-capture what Freud called their lost narcissism.[61] In other words, parents want their children to be sheltered from suffering because they would like to not suffer also. In referring to "his majesty the baby," Freud posited that parents submit to the will of their children so that they can experience, on a vicarious level, the freedom and pleasure that parents have had to give up.[62]

Thus, in an effort to idealize their children so that they can access their own pleasure and freedom through identification, narcissistic parents stop seeing themselves as authority figures and instead focus on keeping their children happy.[63] As Shrier insists, without understanding the structure of narcissism, these contemporary parents turn to books and experts in order to learn how to cater to their children's mental health and happiness: "More than anything, we wanted to raise "happy kids." We looked to the wellness experts for help. We devoured their best-selling parenting books, which established the methods by which we would educate, correct, and even speak to our own children" (xv–xvi). Since parents do not trust their own parenting instincts and they are afraid to do the wrong thing, they turn to outside authorities who may or may not know what they are talking about.[64] Moreover, this reliance on external experts makes the parents self-conscious and full of doubt, which further undermines their ability to provide structure and moral education for their children.

In confusing parenting with therapy, adults apply faulty psychological theories as they eliminate the important roles that rules, limits, and discipline play in human development:

Guided by these experts, we adopted a therapeutic approach to parenting. We learned to offer our kids the reasons behind every rule and request. We never, ever spanked. We perfected the "time-out" and provided thorough explanation for any punishment (which we then rebranded as a "consequence" to remove any associated shame and make us feel less authoritarian). Successful parenting became a function with a single coefficient: our kids' happiness at any given instant. An ideal childhood meant no pain, no discomfort, no fights, no failure – and absolutely no hint of "trauma."

(xvi)

While I do not think we should return to the days of corporal punishment, what has been lost in therapeutic parenting is the role of reality testing and rule enforcement. Many young people are growing up without an accurate understanding of their personal strengths and weaknesses, and this lack of judgment is coupled with a sense that shared rules and standards do not apply to them.[65] Since parents are so afraid of traumatizing their children, they refuse to set vital limits, and when young people show up on college campuses, they are not only riddled by self-doubt and dependency, but they also think that their schools should serve as surrogate parents.

The Parenting-Therapeutic Complex

As Shrier documents, parents are not only acting as amateur therapists for their children, but they are also turning to mental health practitioners in order to diagnose and medicate these young people:

> The more closely we examined our kids, the more glaring their deviations from an endless array of benchmarks – academic, speech, social and emotional. Each now felt like catastrophe. We rushed our kids back to the mental health professionals who had guided our parenting, this time for testing, diagnosis, counseling, and medication. We needed our kids and everyone around them to know: our kids weren't shy, they had "social anxiety disorder" or "social phobia." They weren't poorly behaved, they had "oppositional defiant disorder." They weren't disruptive students, they had "ADHD." It wasn't our fault, and it wasn't theirs. We would attack and finally eliminate the stigma surrounding these diagnoses. Rates at which our children received them soared.
>
> (xvi)

In the passage, Shrier offers an important insight regarding why parents may want their children to have a psychiatric diagnosis: By saying that their kids have a mental disease, parents are able to free themselves from any blame or responsibility regarding their children's poor mental health.[66] If their children can be given an accepted diagnostic label, they have a clear identity, and everything can be blamed on faulty genes and neurotransmitters or some external traumatic event.

In terms of narcissistic parents, a key feature of this psychopathology is the fear of any criticism; since the main drive is to have the good self recognized by others, any real or imagined criticism is perceived as a direct threat to the ideal ego.[67] Parents, then, who see their children as suffering from bad genes, can escape any personal responsibility, and there are many individuals and corporations that feed off of this desire for a medical explanation for human discontent.[68] As we have seen, when a diagnosis does not lead to medication, there is often a whole host of therapies that can provide a mode of substitute parenting.

Shrier adds that "expert diagnoses often altered kids' perceptions of themselves" (xvii). In other words, some children and young adults not only seek out a diagnosis to gain a stable sense of identity and meaning, but when they are given a diagnosis, they start to see themselves through the lens of a disorder.[69] Making matters worse is that all levels of education have started to diagnose and accommodate young people starting at an early age: "School mental health staffs expanded: more psychologists, more counselors, more social workers. The new regime would diagnose and accommodate, not punish or reward. It directed kids in routinized habits of monitoring and sharing their bad feelings. It trained teachers to understand "trauma" as the root of student misbehavior and academic underperformance" (xvii). From this perspective, the generalized therapeutic culture produces a generalized conception of trauma that results in a replacement of education with bad therapy. Even more concerning, the constant focus on young people's mental health results in over-medicating and under-educating.[70] In centering everyone's attention on the feelings of these young people, a dispersed form of paranoia is developed: Every feeling has to be monitored so that suffering can be avoided, but the result is an increase in perceived discontent and mental illness.

To be clear, my point is not that therapy is in itself bad or that people should not tend to their emotions; rather, we need to provide effective modes of therapeutic intervention for the right people at the right time; we also have to stop confusing therapy with education, parenting, and politics. Furthermore, it is vital to turn to psychoanalysis to understand both individual psychopathologies and effective models of treatment. However, since psychoanalysis is constantly being misunderstood and dismissed, we end up falling back to pre-psychoanalytic understandings of mental health.

Blame the iPhone?

While many cultural critics and psychologists blame new technologies, like the smartphone, for the recent uptake in reported depression and anxiety for young adults, Shrier does not think we can blame many of these issues on technology:

> The source of their problem is not reducible to Instagram or Snapchat. Bosses and teachers report – and young people agree – that members of the rising generation are utterly underprepared to accomplish basic tasks we expect all adults to dispatch: ask for a raise; show up for work during a period of national political strife; show up for work at all; fulfill obligations they undertake without requiring extensive breaks to attend to their "mental health."
>
> (xvii)

From Shrier's perspective, smartphones and social media have not caused the current spike in depression and anxiety; instead, bad therapy and counter-productive parenting have paved the way for young people to turn to media technologies in order to escape from their internal sense of discomfort.[71] Making matters worse is that many social media sites present false models of therapy and diagnosis as impressionable teens seek out a mental health diagnosis so that they can secure a stable identity and become part of a group based on shared suffering.[72]

For Shrier, at the heart of this mental health crisis is a fear of taking risks and being responsible for one's actions: "They are leery of the risks and freedoms that are all but synonymous with growing up" (xviii). Young people appear to be resisting becoming responsible, free adults because they have grown up in a world of hyper-awareness where every thought and feeling has to be scrutinized and monitored.[73] Since parents do not trust these young people to do the right thing on their own, these adults are motivated to step in and control their children on a psychological level: "These kids are lonely. They settle into emotional pain for reasons that seem, even to their parents, a little mysterious. Parents seek answers from mental health experts, and when our kids inevitably receive a diagnosis, they grasp it with pride and relief: a whole life, reduced to a single point" (xviii). On one level, kids are lonely because they spend so much time alone in their rooms staring at their phones and laptops, but they are also isolated because parents are afraid to let them go outside and face the perceived dangers of the external world.[74] Of course, the media has induced people to think that the world is much more dangerous than it actually is since media corporations feed off of fear, yet underlying this relation between young people and media sources is the absence of parents limiting their children's access to these devices.[75]

In response to this heightened media-induced paranoia, young people seek out a diagnosis in order to gain a stable sense of identity and meaning.[76] If they can blame their negative feelings on some mental or physical condition, then they do not have to examine the true nature of their discomfort and confusion. However, as Freud argues in *Civilization and Its Discontent*, the fundamental cause for our mental suffering is the conflict between society and the individual, and this opposition will never be fully resolved.[77] Freud also insisted that it is within the family structure that the individual learns the necessity of sacrificing their own drives and desires for the good of the social order. By internalizing a conscience in the form of a super-ego, young people identify with the morality and ideals of their culture, and if they do not willingly accept this internal censor, the threat of violence (castration) is often used to motivate them to conform out of fear.[78]

The narcissistic way of dealing with this fundamental conflict between society and the individual is to signal one's conformity while also keeping a sense of being exceptional and special. Narcissists want to see themselves as being good, competent people, and they do this by getting others to recognize their goodness and virtue, but they also know that this conformity to social norms undermines any sense of authenticity and freedom, so they learn how to conform in an ironic, contradictory manner.[79] Moreover, while society tells them that they must control their violent and sexual urges, they find a safe way of releasing these drives through fantasy and indirect forms of aggression.[80]

While narcissists want to have their good self recognized by the imagined social Other, hysterics desire to have their suffering recognized and affirmed. For example, when a young person is diagnosed as having an eating disorder, they receive a stable identity, and others are motivated to take care of them.[81] Furthermore, Freud discovered that hysterical symptoms are often derived from imitating the suffering of others, and so they often do not have any real connection to actual physical pain.[82] Since one can identify with the suffering of others through empathy, the sharing of the same negative emotions becomes a form of group solidarity and bonding.[83] Thus, according to psychoanalytic theory, what we are witnessing today is a high rate of hysteria that is being catered to by narcissistic individuals and institutions.

Through the expansion of our definition of trauma, hysteria is also expanded, and so is the narcissistic response: Parents, therapists, and educators are repressing psychoanalysis and being guilted into catering to misunderstood psychopathologies: "Recasting personality variation as a chiaroscuro of dysfunction, the mental health experts trained kids to regard themselves as disordered. The experts operate from the assumption that everyone requires therapy and that everyone is at least a little 'broken'" (xvii). Although Shrier believes the problem is that these young adults are being over-diagnosed, the real issue is that they are being misdiagnosed, and the proposed solutions are also the wrong ones because of the general repression of psychoanalysis. People simply do not understand hysteria and narcissism, and they also lack a comprehension of how to deal with these pathologies.

What Shrier does understand is that many different groups are invested in seeing young people as suffering from mental issues:

> With the charisma of cult leaders, therapeutic experts convinced millions of parents to see their children as challenged. They infused parenting with self-consciousness and fevered insecurity. They conscripted teachers into a therapeutic order of education, which meant treating every child as emotionally damaged. They pushed pediatricians to ask kids as young as eight – who had presented with nothing more than a stomachache – whether they felt their parents might be better off without them. In the face of experts' implacable self-assurance, schools were eager; pediatricians, willing; and parents, unresisting.
>
> (xviii)

In this disorganized conspiracy, parents, therapists, doctors, educators, and psychologists have unknowingly colluded to convince everyone that young adults are sick and damaged by getting many people to focus on negative emotions.[84]

In a very telling moment, Shrier unconsciously reveals her misguided understanding of psychoanalysis when she discusses her own therapy: "She helped me realize that I wasn't so bad. Most things were someone else's fault. Actually, many of the people around me were worse than I'd realized! Together, we diagnosed them freely. Who knew so many of my close relatives had narcissistic personality disorder? I found this solar plexus–level comforting. In quick order, my therapist became a really expensive friend, one who agreed with me about almost everything and liked to talk smack about people we (sort of) knew in common" (4). What is so telling about the passage is that Shrier describes her therapy as a conversation based on providing knowledge and agreement. Instead of the therapist remaining neutral, it appears that the therapist reinforced Shrier's desire for love, recognition, and knowledge; in other words, the therapist fed the transference and fueled her patient's underlying desires.[85] By seeing her therapist as an expensive friend who supported her thoughts and feelings, Shrier fell into the trap of reproducing a narcissistic transference.[86] Not only did her therapist see things her way, but this other also reinforced the patient's aggression by agreeing with her indirect attacks on other people.

My goal here is not to call people names, but we need to have an accurate understanding of different pathologies and how therapy actually can work on a psychoanalytic level. One key difference between most forms of therapy and effective psychoanalysis is that the analyst rarely talks or faces the patient. In order to maintain a position of neutrality, the analyst cannot simply respond to the demands of the patient.[87] The main reason for this neutrality is that the patient has to learn how to speak without self-censoring, and thus, the neutrality of the analyst is supposed to create a space for the neutrality of the patient. Since the goal is to discover new things about oneself, it makes no sense to reinforce current desires, fears, and defense mechanisms.

Another vital aspect of psychoanalysis is working through the transference, which entails the patient no longer seeing the analyst as the one who can save them.[88] Even though people go into treatment to be saved by others, it is this desire to transfer responsibility onto the other that must be acknowledged and then removed. From this perspective, psychoanalysis does provide freedom and responsibility as one learns to rely on oneself to confront and resolve problems. On a basic level, real trauma threatens this process because people who have PTSD cannot symbolize the shocking event that has undermined their sense of mental control.[89] However, as Freud discovered, the way to overcome the repetition of trauma is to slowly learn how to symbolize it and divest from its power.[90] Unfortunately, the new trend is to turn to some form of cognitive behavioral therapy (CBT) to change how people think about their traumas and other emotions, but as we have seen in previous chapters, this form of therapy is often based on transference and hypnotic suggestion. Therefore, instead of working through the dependency on the saving Other, one simply learns to conform to the Other's demands. While Freud started off using a similar type of method, he eventually discovered that it was best for the patient to speak freely without any guidance, which is the opposite of hypnosis and CBT.

Another important feature of psychoanalysis is that it is confidential, and the emphasis is on the singular patient, but what we find in many forms of contemporary therapy is that the neutrality of the patient and freedom of the patient are often compromised by interfering forces. For example, Shrier describes how parents can use therapy to monitor their children: "A few moms told me, in roundabout verbiage, that they had hired a therapist to surveil their surly teen's thoughts and feelings. The therapist doesn't tell me what my daughter says exactly, the moms assured me, but she sort of lets me know everything's okay. And occasionally, I gathered, the therapist relayed to Mom specific information gleaned from the little prisoner of war" (5–6). In this context, therapy acts to enhance the way parents surveil their children.[91]

As Shrier documents, misguided therapy can do more harm than good, but this problem is rarely acknowledged: "Therapy can exacerbate marital stress, compromise a patient's resilience, render a patient more traumatized, more depressed, and undermine her self-efficacy so she's less able to turn her life around. Therapy may lead a patient by degrees – sunk into a leather sofa, well-placed tissue box close at hand – to become overly dependent on her therapist" (8). Since most modes of therapy do not work through the transference, they can end up increasing a person's dependency and also reinforce their negative emotions and thoughts: "Therapy can hijack our normal processes of resilience, interrupting our psyche's ability to heal itself, in its own way, at its own time" (9). Shrier's argument here is that when we get people to focus on their emotions, we can undermine their resilience and prevent them from figuring out things on their own. While this might be true, there is still the need for people to confront their own unconscious desires, fears, and mechanisms, and this cannot be done with a reflecting therapist or friend. The problem, then, is not that we rely too much on therapy; the issue is that most therapy is counter-productive.

In discussing her own therapy, Shrier laments how it pushed her to focus on her own suffering: "I remembered saving up emotional injuries to report to my therapist so that we would have something to talk about at our session – injuries I might have just let go" (9). This type of hysterical transference places the therapist in the position of the one who knows, cares about, and recognizes the patient's suffering, but one of the goals of analysis is to expose the underlying desire for love, recognition, and knowledge, and this occurs through the patient's own thoughts concerning the transfer of responsibility onto the idealized analyst.[92] If this underlying desire for transference is not exposed, then it continues to feed hysterical suffering.

Since Shrier appears to have no understanding of psychoanalysis, she tends to present a misguided notion of how therapy works: "Interestingly, even when patients' symptoms are made objectively worse by therapy, they tend to assume the therapy has helped. We rely largely on how "purged" we feel when we leave a therapist's office to justify our sense that the therapy is working. We rarely track objective markers, for example, the state of our career or relationships, before reaching a conclusion" (9). It is clear that Shrier believes that therapy should be judged by how well a patient adapts to social demands, but this conception does nothing to help people to explore their own inner minds as they become free to make decisions based on their accurate assessment of external reality. In fact, much of Lacan's early work concerns critiquing American ego psychology and the focus on adapting to social expectations.[93] After all, a defining aspect of obsessional neurosis and narcissism is the desire to comply with the desires of others.

Shrier's repression of psychoanalysis is evident in her discussion of the ineffectiveness of most forms of therapy: "while some therapies have shown success in circumscribed areas – like cognitive behavioral therapy has in treating phobias – those who study the efficacy of therapies often point out that the results across treatment types are not terribly impressive" (11). The truth is that there is ample evidence that only psychoanalysis has sustained, long-term benefits for most mental disorders, but since so many people have a negative and prejudiced feeling about this mode of therapy, they often turn to CBT and medication as the only possible solutions.[94] In fact, Shrier dismisses Freud and psychoanalysis by isolating hysteria from the distant past: "Therapists induced an epidemic of the phony ailment neurasthenia at the start of the twentieth century" (11). Instead of realizing that we now have a major increase in hysterical symptoms, Shrier simply blames psychoanalysis for producing fake psycho-somatic disorders. Since she does not know that hysteria is defined by the use of real and imagined suffering to gain identity and to manipulate others on an unconscious level, she fails to see how the recent increase in depression and anxiety is related to the narcissistic accommodation of hysteria.

From Shrier's cynical perspective, what is really driving the focus on trauma and therapy inside and outside of higher education is the fact that therapist have a financial incentive to keep patients by not trying to cure them: "Shrinks are badly incentivized where iatrogenesis is concerned. A doctor may decide that a patient would no longer benefit from thyroid medication, discontinue it, and keep the patient. A therapist gets paid by the dose. Once she decides you don't need therapy, she loses a customer" (12). Although it is possible that some therapists and psychiatrists do depend on keeping their patients unwell, the bigger problem is that there is little consensus concerning the causes and solutions to specific mental disorders.

Return to Technology

Even though Shrier does not want to blame technology for the rise in reported anxiety and depression, she does affirm that new modes of social media cater to the relationship between hysteria and narcissism: "Teenage communication today is more constant, largely digital, and, even among teen girls, far more superficial than it was a generation ago. Less baring of souls, more trading of memes. Even to their best friends, they communicate only this: that they are going through something bad and serious, something that will require their friends' sympathy and indulgence" (16). It is difficult to determine how much young people are changing how they communicate with their peers, but what Shrier gets right is that people often express their suffering in order to gain the sympathy of the people around them, yet what she leaves out is that this type of relationship between the expression of hysterical symptoms and the empathy of a narcissistic or hysterical audience occurs mainly on an unconscious level.[95]

Like most contemporary therapists and psychologists, what Shrier does not grasp is that the unconscious is caused by repression, and repression is derived from self-deception based on the desire to escape feelings of guilt, shame, and responsibility.[96] In order to maintain this type of repression, it is necessary to blame others, the past, or biology for one's problems and discontent. When friends, parents, educators, and therapists merely affirm the suffering subject's complaints, repressions are reinforced. In the case of hysterical empathy, people identify with the suffering of others, and this enables them the ability to participate in a victim complex.[97] In contrast, when others try not only to empathize but resolve and heal the suffering, they are often motivated by a narcissistic desire to represent themselves as being good. None of these reactions help people to discover the root causes of their suffering.

As Shrier reports, many young adults feel that they have been abused and trau-matized, but even if some of them may be exaggerating, friends simply affirm their complaints because they want to maintain their relationship: "Some of her friends complain their parents are 'emotionally abusive,' but when I ask Nora why their therapists haven't called Child Services, she seems unperturbed. Yes, she assumes they're sort of exaggerating. To preserve the friendship, you suspend disbelief" (16). Since people who express their suffering want to have their pain recognized by others, it is understandable that friends do not question the source or the severity of the problem; in fact, one of the effects of the victim complex is to eliminate all criticism or questioning, but it is unclear how people can escape this destructive dynamic through sympathy and empathy.

This issue of how to respond to the hysterical complaint is a key issue for therapy and psychoanalysis because one does not want simply to dismiss the expression of suffering, but one also does not want to reinforce it.[98] The psychoanalytic solution is to allow the suffering person to speak without censorship and without the analyst being empathic. By not responding to the underlying desire for love, recognition, and knowledge, the analyst helps the patient to discover, on their own, the desires that underlie particular demands. As Lacan demonstrates, when a child asks a parent for something, they are not just demanding a particular object – they are desiring uncon-ditional love, recognition, and knowledge.[99] This drive to receive the empathy of the other can result in the production of a transference where one relies on being saved by the idealized Other. Moreover, this Other represents the ego ideal, which Freud ties to passionate love, hypnosis, and the formation of armies, churches, and political rallies.[100] In other words, at the heart of social groups, we find a relationship where someone transfers responsibility and power onto some idealized person or ideology. In this escape from responsibility and freedom, all guilt and shame can be avoided, but the cost is a loss of independence and reality testing.

In the case of hysteria and narcissism, the complete submission to the idealized Other is avoided by transforming the Other into a neutral audience void of any power or control. A problem, then, for psychoanalysis is how the analyst remains neutral if this neutrality can be used by the neurotic patient as a form of safe vali-dation. Lacan's great contribution to this problem concerns his use of different techniques to undermine the neutralization of the analyst while still allowing the analyst to be neutral.[101] One key innovation was to stop ending each session after 50 minutes, and instead, he started to vary the time of each meeting.[102] While the patient may respond to this type of "punctuation" by giving it some specific mean-ing, Lacan's main point is that the analyst's desire must always remain undefined, and the analyst should do nothing to feed the desire of the patient to place the ana-lyst in the position of the one who is supposed to know.

For many therapists and analysts, it is absurd to ask them not to try to understand or care about their patients, but what drives this desire to be the one who knows and cares may be a narcissistic desire to see oneself as being good. By having the ideal ego recognized by others, the narcissist is able to maintain a positive self-image, but this form of relationship is reliant on removing all power and desire from the other. In the context of some forms of therapy, the therapist uses the patient as a blank screen to reflect the therapist's own thoughts and feelings; meanwhile, the suffering subject uses the therapist simply to verify and reflect their own desires. In what Lacan called the trap of imaginary duality, nothing really changes since any new or discomforting unconscious material is repressed through a process of narcissistic reflection.[103]

As I have been arguing, since psychoanalysis has itself been repressed by mental health practitioners, the result is an increase in reported student issues coupled with an increase in ineffective therapies:

> Forty-two percent of the rising generation currently has a mental health diagnosis, rendering "normal" increasingly abnormal. One in six US children aged two to eight years old has a diagnosed mental, behavioral, or developmental disorder. More than 10 percent of American kids have an ADHD diagnosis – double the expected prevalence rate based on population surveys in other countries. Nearly 10 percent of kids now have a diagnosed anxiety disorder. Teens today so profoundly identify with these diagnoses, they display them in social media profiles, alongside a picture and family name.
>
> (17)

In response to this mental health "crisis," people have to learn that many people receive a "secondary gain" from expressing their suffering, but the causes for this mode of hysteria is largely unconscious.[104] Moreover, the solution is not simply to give them drugs or reinforce their symptoms; we need to find ways to change the social understanding of these problems as we provide psychoanalytic treatment for more people.

One place to start concerns the way trauma is now being defined by educators, parents, and therapists: "It seems perfectly reasonable to talk about a child's 'trauma' from the death of a pet or the routine humiliation of being picked last for a sports team" (19). In this expansion of how people define trauma, all sense of proportionality has been lost. However, it is hard to discuss this problem because it looks like victim-blaming.[105] Yet, as Shrier documents, we continue to spend more money on therapy as a society, but the rates of reported mental health issues continue to increase: "And yet as treatments for anxiety and depression have become more sophisticated and more readily available, adolescent anxiety and depression have ballooned" (20). The problem is not only are people being over-diagnosed and over-medicated, but the people who need help are getting the wrong types of help. Before I outline some of the main ways to try to fix the college mental health crisis, I want to examine in the next chapter why and how universities are being placed in the position of substitute parents.

Notes

1 Brothers, Doris, and Jon Sletvold. *A New Vision of Psychoanalytic Theory, Practice and Supervision: Talking Bodies*. Routledge, 2023.
2 Shrier, Abigail. *Bad Therapy: Why the Kids Aren't Growing Up*. Swift Press, 2024.

3 Freud, Sigmund. "On beginning the treatment (further recommendations on the technique of psycho-analysis I)." *Standard Edition* 12 (1913): 121–144.
4 Lacan, Jacques, Alan Sheridan, and Malcolm Bowie. "The direction of the treatment and the principles of its power 1." *Écrits: A Selection*. Routledge, 2020, 250–310.
5 Thompson, M. Guy. "Freud's conception of neutrality." *Contemporary Psychoanalysis* 32.1 (1996): 25–42.
6 Malin, Barnet D. "Kohut and Lacan: mirror opposites." *Psychoanalytic Inquiry* 31.1 (2011): 58–74.
7 Diatkine, Gilbert. "Lacan and the transference." *The International Journal of Psychoanalysis* 104.4 (2023): 722–736.
8 Lacan, Jacques, Alan Sheridan, and Malcolm Bowie. "The function and field of speech and language in psychoanalysis." *Écrits: A Selection*. Routledge, 2020, 33–125.
9 Willemsen, Hessel. "Early trauma and affect: The importance of the body for the development of the capacity to symbolize." *Journal of Analytical Psychology* 59.5 (2014): 695–712.
10 Yehuda, Rachel, and Amy Lehrner. "Intergenerational transmission of trauma effects: Putative role of epigenetic mechanisms." *World Psychiatry* 17.3 (2018): 243–257.
11 Zahavi, Dan. "Empathy and mirroring: Husserl and Gallese." *Life, Subjectivity & Art: Essays in Honor of Rudolf Bernet*. Dordrecht: Springer Netherlands, 2011, 217–254.
12 Hutman, Ted, and Mirella Dapretto. "The emergence of empathy during infancy." *Cognition, Brain, Behavior* 13.4 (2009): 367.
13 Baker, Howard S., and Margaret N. Baker. "Heinz Kohut's self psychology: An overview." *The American Journal of Psychiatry* 144.1 (1987): 1–9.
14 Hamburg, Paul. "Interpretation and empathy: Reading Lacan with Kohut." *The International Journal of Psycho-Analysis* 72.2 (1991): 347.
15 Muller, John P. "Ego and subject in Lacan." *Psychoanalytic Review* 69.2 (1982): 234.
16 Lacan, Jacques. "The seminar of Jacques Lacan: Book VIII: Transference: 1960–1961." *Polity Press* (2017).
17 Freud, Sigmund. "The history of the psychoanalytic movement." *The Psychoanalytic Review (1913–1957)* 3 (1916): 406.
18 Freud, Sigmund. *Dora: An Analysis of a Case of Hysteria*. Simon and Schuster, 1997.
19 Dick, Kirby, and Amy Ziering. *The Hunting Ground: The Inside Story of Sexual Assault on American College Campuses*. Simon and Schuster, 2016.
20 Krebs, Christopher P., et al. "Comparing sexual assault prevalence estimates obtained with direct and indirect questioning techniques." *Violence Against Women* 17.2 (2011): 219–235.
21 Javorka, McKenzie, and Rebecca Campbell. "'This isn't just a police issue': Tensions between criminal justice and university responses to sexual assault among college students." *American Journal of Community Psychology* 67.1–2 (2021): 152–165.
22 Wilson, Mitchell. "The analyst as listening-accompanist: Desire in Bion and Lacan." *The Psychoanalytic Quarterly* 87.2 (2018): 237–264.
23 Bloom, Paul. *Against Empathy: The Case for Rational Compassion*. Random House, 2017.
24 Marshall, Jocelyn E. "Not letting it go: Anger, empathy, and interdisciplinarity as trauma-informed approach." *Trauma-Informed Pedagogy: Addressing Gender-Based Violence in the Classroom*. Emerald Publishing Limited, 2022, 157–171.
25 Elliott, Raymond Kenneth. "Imagination: 'A kind of magical faculty'." *Study of Education Pb*. Routledge, 2018, 248–264.
26 Elliott, Raymond Kenneth. "Imagination: 'A kind of magical faculty'." *Study of Education Pb*. Routledge, 2018, 248–264.
27 Freud, Sigmund. *Totem and Taboo*. Routledge, 2012.
28 Kanaan, Richard A. A. "Freud's hysteria and its legacy." *Handbook of Clinical Neurology* 139 (2016): 37–44.
29 Muller, John. "Lacan's mirror stage." *Psychoanalytic Inquiry* 5.2 (1985): 233–252.

30 Freud, Sigmund. *Group Psychology and the Analysis of the Ego*. WW Norton & Company, 1975.
31 Hickok, Gregory. *The Myth of Mirror Neurons: The Real Neuroscience of Communication and Cognition*. WW Norton & Company, 2014.
32 Samuels, Robert. *The Psychoanalytic Understanding of Consciousness, Free Will, Language, and Reason: What Makes Us Human?* Routledge, 2023.
33 Shweder, Richard A., et al. "Likeness and likelihood in everyday thought: Magical thinking in judgments about personality [and comments and reply]." *Current Anthropology* 18.4 (1977): 637–658.
34 Samuels, Robert, and Robert Samuels. "Damasio's error: The politics of biological determinism after Freud." *Psychoanalyzing the Politics of the New Brain Sciences*. Springer, 2017, 9–33.
35 Menaker, Esther. "The self-image as defense and resistance." *The Psychoanalytic Quarterly* 29.1 (1960): 72–81.
36 Hayne, Harlene, Maryanne Garry, and Elizabeth F. Loftus. "On the continuing lack of scientific evidence for repression." *Behavioral and Brain Sciences* 29.5 (2006): 521–522.
37 McGuire, Michael T. "Repression, resistance, and recall of the past: Some reconsiderations." *The Psychoanalytic Quarterly* 39.3 (1970): 427–448.
38 Bainbridge, Alan, and Linden West. *Psychoanalysis and Education: Minding a Gap*. Routledge, 2018.
39 Kaplan, Cora. "Fictions of feminism: Figuring the maternal." *Feminist Studies* 1 (Spring 1994): 153–167.
40 Ragland-Sullivan, Ellie. "The paternal metaphor: A Lacanian theory of language." *Revue Internationale de Philosophie* (1992): 49–92.
41 Sprengnether, Madelon. "Feminist criticism and psychoanalysis." *A History of Feminist Literary Criticism* (2007): 235–263.
42 Samuels, Robert. *Teaching the Rhetoric of Resistance: The Popular Holocaust and Social Change in a Post-9/11 World*. Springer, 2007.
43 Richmond, Sarah. "Magic in Sartre's early philosophy." *Reading Sartre*. Routledge, 2010, 155–170.
44 Rensmann, Lars. *The Politics of Unreason: The Frankfurt School and the Origins of Modern Antisemitism*. Suny Press, 2017.
45 Wolin, Richard. *The Seduction of Unreason: The Intellectual Romance with Fascism from Nietzsche to Postmodernism*. Princeton University Press, 2019.
46 Prinz, Jesse. "Against empathy." *The Southern Journal of Philosophy* 49 (2011): 214–233.
47 Krizan, Zlatan, and Omesh Johar. "Envy divides the two faces of narcissism." *Journal of personality* 80.5 (2012): 1415–1451.
48 Fenigstein, Allan. "Paranoia and self-focused attention." *The Self in European and North American Culture: Development and Processes*. Dordrecht: Springer Netherlands, 1995, 183–192.
49 Zhang, Irene Y., Deborah M. Powell, and Silvia Bonaccio. "The role of fear of negative evaluation in interview anxiety and social-evaluative workplace anxiety." *International Journal of Selection and Assessment* 30.2 (2022): 302–310.
50 Schutzman, Mady. *The Aesthetics of Hysteria: Performance, Pathology, and Advertising*. New York University, 1994.
51 Scott, Graham G., et al. "Posting photos on Facebook: The impact of narcissism, social anxiety, loneliness, and shyness." *Personality and Individual Differences* 133 (2018): 67–72.
52 Vescovelli, Francesca, et al. "University counseling service for improving students' mental health." *Psychological Services* 14.4 (2017): 470.
53 Shrier, Abigail. *Bad Therapy: Why the Kids Aren't Growing Up*. Swift Press, 2024.

54 Sapadin, Kate, and Beth L. G. Hollander. "Distinguishing the need for crisis mental health services among college students." *Psychological Services* 19.2 (2022): 317.
55 Keller, Heidi, et al. "Cultural orientations and historical changes as predictors of parenting behaviour." *International Journal of Behavioral Development* 29.3 (2005): 229–237.
56 Lipson, Sarah Ketchen, Emily G. Lattie, and Daniel Eisenberg. "Increased rates of mental health service utilization by US college students: 10-year population-level trends (2007–2017)." *Psychiatric Services* 70.1 (2019): 60–63.
57 Cui, Ming, et al. "Indulgent parenting, helicopter parenting, and well-being of parents and emerging adults." *Journal of Child and Family Studies* 28 (2019): 860–871.
58 Pinker, Steven. "Enlightenment now, the case for reason, science, humanism, and progress." *Revista Española de Investigaciones Sociológicas (REIS)* 170.170 (2020): 163–167.
59 Campbell, Bradley, and Jason Manning. "The rise of victimhood culture." *Microaggressions, Safe Spaces, and the New Culture Wars, the Rise of Victimhood Culture: Microaggressions, Safe Spaces, and the New Culture Wars* 1 (2018): 265.
60 Bertolote, José Manoel, and Alexandra Fleischmann. "Suicide and psychiatric diagnosis: A worldwide perspective." *World Psychiatry* 1.3 (2002): 181.
61 Freud, Sigmund. *On Narcissism: An Introduction.* Read Books Ltd, 2014.
62 Shulman, Michael. "Teaching Freud's 'on narcissism'." *American Imago* 75.2 (2018): 297–302.
63 Elkind, David. "Instrumental narcissism in parents." *Bulletin of the Menninger Clinic* 55.3 (1991): 299.
64 Lasch, Christopher. "The culture of narcissism." *American Social Character.* Routledge, 2019, 241–267.
65 Layton, Lynne. "Grandiosity, neoliberalism, and neoconservatism." *Psychoanalytic Inquiry* 34.5 (2014): 463–474.
66 Harborne, Alexandra, Miranda Wolpert, and Linda Clare. "Making sense of ADHD: A battle for understanding? Parents' views of their children being diagnosed with ADHD." *Clinical Child Psychology and Psychiatry* 9.3 (2004): 327–339.
67 Derry, Kate L., Jeneva L. Ohan, and Donna M. Bayliss. "Fearing failure: Grandiose narcissism, vulnerable narcissism, and emotional reactivity in children." *Child Development* 91.3 (2020): e581–e596.
68 Samuels, Robert, and Robert Samuels. "Drugging discontent: Psychoanalysis, drives, and the governmental university medical pharmaceutical complex (GUMP)." *Psychoanalyzing the Politics of the New Brain Sciences.* Springer, 2017, 115–136.
69 Lafrance, Michelle N., and Suzanne McKenzie-Mohr. "The DSM and its lure of legitimacy." *Feminism & Psychology* 23.1 (2013): 119–140.
70 Watkins, Lance Vincent, and Heather Angus-Leppan. "Increasing incidence of autism spectrum disorder: Are we over-diagnosing?" *Advances in Autism* 9.1 (2022): 42–52.
71 Twenge, Jean M., et al. "Worldwide increases in adolescent loneliness." *Journal of Adolescence* 93 (2021): 257–269.
72 Dewak, Hadil. *Scrolling for a Diagnosis: The Effects of Self-Diagnosing Content on Social Media on Young Adults' Mental Health.* BS thesis. University of Twente, 2023.
73 Muris, Peter, et al. "Monitoring and anxiety disorders symptoms in children." *Personality and Individual Differences* 29.4 (2000): 775–781.
74 Skenazy, Lenore. *Free-Range Kids, How to Raise Safe, Self-Reliant Children (Without Going Nuts with Worry).* John Wiley & Sons, 2009.
75 Schmuck, Desiree, et al. "Out of control? How parents' perceived lack of control over children's smartphone use affects children's self-esteem over time." *New Media & Society* 25.1 (2023): 199–219.
76 Altheide, David L. "The news media, the problem frame, and the production of fear." *The Sociological Quarterly* 38.4 (1997): 647–668.

77 Freud, Sigmund. *Civilization and Its Discontents-Freud*. Lebooks Editora, 2024.
78 Calogeras, Roy C., and Fabian X. Schupper. "Origins and early formulations of the Oedipus complex." *Journal of the American Psychoanalytic Association* 20.4 (1972): 751–775.
79 Samuels, Robert. "(Liberal) narcissism." *Routledge Handbook of Psychoanalytic Political Theory*. Routledge, 2019, 151–161.
80 Russell, Gillian A. "Narcissism and the narcissistic personality disorder: A comparison of the theories of Kernberg and Kohut." *British Journal of Medical Psychology* 58.2 (1985): 137–148.
81 Leonidas, Carolina, and Manoel Antônio dos Santos. "Symbiotic Illusion and female identity construction in eating disorders: A psychoanalytical psychosomatics' perspective." *Ágora: Estudos em Teoria Psicanalítica* 23 (2020): 84–93.
82 Campbell, Jan. "Hysteria, mimesis and the phenomenological imaginary." *Textual Practice* 19.3 (2005): 331–351.
83 Pigman, George W. "Freud and the history of empathy." *The International Journal of Psycho-Analysis* 76.2 (1995): 237.
84 Finn, Janet L., and Lynn Nybell. "Introduction: Capitalizing on concern: The making of troubled children and troubling youth in late capitalism." *Childhood* 8.2 (2001): 139–145.
85 Corradi, Richard B. "A conceptual model of transference and its psychotherapeutic application." *Journal of the American Academy of Psychoanalysis and Dynamic Psychiatry* 34.3 (2006): 415–439.
86 Boadella, David. "Transference, politics, and narcissism." *International Journal of Psychotherapy* 4.3 (1999).
87 Hoffer, Axel. "Toward a definition of psychoanalytic neutrality." *Journal of the American Psychoanalytic Association* 33.4 (1985): 771–795.
88 Freud, Sigmund. "The dynamics of transference." *Classics in Psychoanalytic Techniques* 12 (1912): 97–108.
89 Gil, Sharon. "Is secondary traumatization a negative therapeutic response?" *Journal of Loss and Trauma* 20.5 (2015): 410–416.
90 Freud, Sigmund. "Mourning and melancholia." *The Standard Edition of the Complete Psychological Works of Sigmund Freud 14.1914–1916*. Random House, 2001, 237–258.
91 Robinson, Brittany A., et al. "Social context, parental monitoring, and multisystemic therapy outcomes." *Psychotherapy* 52.1 (2015): 103.
92 Talero, Maria. "Temporality and the therapeutic subject: The phenomenology of transference, remembering, and working-through." *Rereading Freud: Psychoanalysis through Philosophy* (2004): 165–179.
93 Lacan, Jacques. *The Ego in Freud's Theory and in the Technique of Psychoanalysis, 1954–1955*. Vol. 2. WW Norton & Company, 1988.
94 Smit, Yolba, et al. "The effectiveness of long-term psychoanalytic psychotherapy – A meta-analysis of randomized controlled trials." *Clinical Psychology Review* 32.2 (2012): 81–92.
95 Sennett, Richard. "Narcissism and modern culture." *October* (1977): 70–79.
96 Joseph, Rhawn. "Awareness, the origin of thought, and the role of conscious self-deception in resistance and repression." *Psychological Reports* 46.3 (1980): 767–781.
97 Samuels, Robert, and Robert Samuels. "Pathos, Hysteria, and the left." *Zizek and the Rhetorical Unconscious: Global Politics, Philosophy, and Subjectivity*. Springer, 2020, 33–47.
98 Pepeli, Hara. "Psychoanalysis: A treatment, a cure . . . or much more than that." *Journal of the Centre for Freudian Analysis and Research* 13 (2003).
99 Ahmadzadeh, Shideh. "The study of desire: A Lacanian perspective." *Teaching English Language* 1.2 (2007): 139–153.

100 Freud, Sigmund. *Group Psychology and the Analysis of the Ego.* WW Norton & Company, 1975.
101 Ouvry, Olivier. "Interpretation and equivocation." *Research in Psychoanalysis* 1 (2018): 66–73.
102 Pietrusza, Celeste, and Derek Hook. "'You're kicking me out?' Scansion and the variable-length session in Lacanian clinical praxis." *Psychodynamic Practice* 22.2 (2016): 102–119.
103 Lacan, Jacques, Alan Sheridan, and Malcolm Bowie. "Aggressivity in psychoanalysis." *Écrits: A Selection.* Routledge, 2020, 9–32.
104 van Egmond, Jacques J. "Multiple meanings of secondary gain." *The American Journal of Psychoanalysis* 63 (2003): 137–147.
105 Conaway, Elizabeth. "Victim blaming." *Entries* (2017): 51.

Chapter 7

The University as a False Family

To further examine the college mental health crisis, I turn to Matthew Bowker's *A Dangerous Place to Be: Identity, Conflict, and Trauma in Higher Education*, which makes the provocative argument that many of the causes for student suffering and ineffective institutional responses stem from the idea that people are treating universities as substitute families.[1] Moreover, Bowker believes that the type of family dynamics being projected onto these schools derives from a fundamental fear that parents have regarding their children's desires and impulses.

A Rejection of the Students' Inner Life

Bowker begins his analysis by claiming that what is driving the crisis in college mental health is a fundamental repression of the subjectivity of the students: "What makes the link between identity and university-based conflict difficult to see is that most controversies have been marked by efforts to ignore or disguise experiences in individuals' inner worlds and to insist on the importance of groups, group identities, and group fantasies about victimization that offer collective ("social") defenses" (ix–x). From this perspective, the problem is not that we are focusing too much on students' self-reported suffering. The issue is that we are focused on group identities and not individual subjectivity.[2]

For Bowker, the focus of our therapeutic attention should be on how families either encourage or block a young person's quest for identity and attachment: "For the individual, this struggle begins in the family and in the home, where attachments to and interactions with significant others either foster or impede the work of shaping an identity that is rooted in self-contact and suitable for life in civil society" (x). From this perspective, a key to human development is the way identity and relationships are formed, and families represent the main source of this development.[3] Furthermore, he ties the formation of personal identity to an individual's sense of meaning and value: "It is necessary to know that we matter to others in order to secure the feeling that we matter to ourselves" (x). In focusing on how individuals perceive the ways they are valued by others, Bowker tends to concentrate on self-esteem and not the development of reality testing and drive control. In

DOI: 10.4324/9781003545668-7

other words, the risk of this psychological theory is that it can cater to the narcissism and drive impulses of the isolated individual.

Bowker's major thesis is that parents and other caregivers over-protect their children because they believe that these young people are inherently bad:

> Families and caregivers operating under the assumption that the child's self is "bad" will offer what might be called "inappropriate forms of protection," inasmuch as these protections do not protect the child from demands for adaptation, but, rather, "protect" the child from herself. In lieu of being herself, the child is offered or ascribed a false self, one typically associated with family "pride," which operates as a defense against unconscious identification with the bad self. This inappropriate form of protection, then, condemns the child not only to shame but to profound confusion about her real self, about who she really is and who she might be.
>
> (xii)

According to this theory, parents want their children to conform to some ideal standard of behavior, and when these young people fail to conform, the parents label them as being bad; in other words, in response to this badness, the parents seek to protect the children from their anti-social impulses.[4] In turn, the child responds to this labeling by seeing himself as a false self while still identifying on an unconscious level with a sense of being bad.[5]

This theory does incorporate different psychoanalytic concepts, but what is missing from this account is the narcissism of the parents and the unconscious hysteria of the children.[6] As we have seen, parents want to idealize their children because they want to identify with this idealization, and they also desire to be seen as being good and competent by protecting their children and affirming their wishes, feelings, and demands.[7] The problem is not, then, that they see their children as being bad; the issue often is that they want to see them as being good, and so they repress the anti-social nature of all human beings.

According to Bowker's thesis, just as a child seeks to be protected from their own badness by over-involved parents, they expect the same thing to happen when they go to college:

> As the child matures, he may come to expect or demand inappropriate forms of care and inappropriate forms of protection from the groups and organizations of which he is a part, particularly if those organizations present themselves as facsimiles of his family home. He will expect these organizations to concur with the fantasies and defenses erected early in life and relied on throughout maturation, since these fantasies and defenses have helped to prevent him from knowing what he suspects to be true about his self: that it is bad, shameful, and unworthy of love.
>
> (xiii)

The idea here is that students want institutions of higher education to act as protective parents who will protect them from their own sense of shame.[8] Although it is clear that parents do seek to get their children to control their anti-social impulses, often by making them feel guilty about their violent and sexual impulses, shame is derived from a feeling that one has not lived up to the standards of the ideal ego.[9] Moreover, from Freud's perspective, the sense that one is not worthy of love is often tied to the internalization of the super-ego through a process of identifying with the morality and aggression of an external authority.[10] In grouping shame, guilt, and a fear of losing love together, Bowker's theory does not fully articulate how these different stages of development relate and differentiate.

While I do agree that institutions of higher education are often asked to take on the role of the family, the reasons behind this demand may not be to protect young people from their own perceived badness; instead, we see a hysterical desire to have suffering recognized and tended to by narcissistic adults who want to feel good about themselves by playing the role of the good, maternal figure.[11] Although Bowker does not recognize this dynamic, he does realize that both the students and the adults are being shaped by unconscious fantasies:

> The more, then, that a university takes on the look, feel, and functions of a family home where inappropriate forms of care were the rule, the more it blurs the line between past and present, between reality, memory, and fantasy, and between life in the family and life outside. The more a university presents itself as a family home for students, the more it encourages students to demand from it a form of care associated not with the feeling of security in being, but with "protection" from the desire to express the self authentically. In other words, the university will protect its members from the presence of their selves.
>
> (xii)

Bowker's thesis here is that what students really want from their universities is to be protected from their own desire to express themselves in an authentic way.[12] I think the problem with this view is that it does not fully grasp the structure of narcissism, which entails conformity with the expectations of others coupled with a desire to be treated as special and unique. The quest for authenticity is not being repressed because one is afraid of it: Authentic self-expression is being blocked because it is in conflict with the demands of socialization.[13]

Grade Obsession and Capitalism

My thesis is that many students seek the empathy of the university because they want to find meaning and identity through expressed suffering. Since they have been told that everyone has been traumatized, they seek recognition, protection, and affirmation from the adults around them.[14] Moreover, they have grown up with a mode of social media that often rewards people for exposing their pain, and they have often been catered to by parents who see it as their role to affirm these expressed symptoms. I think that Bowker misses this underlying hysterical pathology because he combines self-psychology and object relations theory to repress psychoanalysis. By combining together a notion of the authentic self with primitive fantasies concerning the relationship with others, he ends up claiming that students and colleges collude to protect against individual drives and desires: "And the more those in the university identify with students' false selves and engage in comparable defenses against contact with their own original vitality, the more the university will collude with the work of the family to suppress or hide the child's – now the student's – true self, no matter how much emphasis is placed on the student's 'safety'" (xiii). In contrast to this theory of protecting students against their own vitality and authenticity, what we really see is that these institutions often feed the selfish pursuit of pleasure and reward through a capitalistic notion of education.[15] In fact, students are trained at a very young age to compete for grades, but they are not socialized to respect learning for learning's sake; instead, grades represent a form of capital that students pursue on an individual basis.[16] Even if students do not really care about what they are learning, they still often seek to gain a reward by conforming to the expectations of teachers, and this conformity is a cynical and opportunistic attempt to feed the drive to access scarce resources.[17]

Schools, then, socialize students to be borderline sociopaths who only care about gaining grades, credits, and degrees that they can use for their own future benefit.[18] While receiving high grades can feed their narcissistic desire to be seen as good and competent by others, underlying this quest to have the ideal ego verified, we find the self-destructive addiction to exchange value in the form of desiring what others desire.[19] At the center of the Neoliberal education system is this training of young people to only care about external rewards and not their own internal values, so it is unfair then to turn around and blame them for conforming to the system that is reinforced through rewards and punishment.[20] Furthermore, parents buy into this system because they believe that the only way a person can have a successful life is if they do well in school starting at a very young age, and while levels of education do correlate with levels of wealth, the entire system feeds an anti-social pathology.[21]

One reason, then, why students may feel fake and inauthentic is that they are being motivated to conform to a system that combines the pursuit of personal pleasure with the destruction of the self.[22] Like all modes of addiction, what may start off as looking like the individual focusing on their own stimulation and access to desired objects ends up being both self-destructive and anti-social.[23] At the same time, then, that parents encourage students to pursue high grades, they also seek to shame them for being selfish and dominated by their impulses. Likewise, universities not only feed this grade obsession, but they also both celebrate and condemn student enjoyment.[24] On the one hand, these institutions want to see themselves as focusing on learning, but they pour money into student entertainment and services in order to keep present students happy and to attract new high-paying students.[25] One of the results of this process is that many students go into debt while education becomes less of a priority.[26]

Instead of students and faculty focusing on the way grades undermine education and render students obsessed and dissatisfied, the emphasis is often on how they have been victimized by the past or some type of systemic oppression:

> For the adult, or young adult, there can be both real, present-time experiences of victimization and oppression, and experiences interpreted in this way because of

the power of internal dramas to guide, shape, or fit experiences into familiar schemas. In the university, both possibilities are in play and it is difficult, if not impossible, to determine the balance of the two in any given circumstance. Because of this, students' accounts of having been victimized, oppressed, or traumatized should neither be dismissed simply as aspects of fantasy life, nor accepted simply as reality-based accounts of contemporary experience. They may fall into either category, or, more likely, they may represent a mixture of the two.

(xiv)

Bowker makes the important argument here that we need to treat claims of victimization as combining real and imagined threats, but as Freud insists in relation to hysteria, we also have to consider how suffering is used to gain identity and meaning while one employs expressed suffering to influence others.[27] Not only do students often use real and imagined health issues to ask for accommodations, but their commitment to different political causes can be based on an empathic identification with the suffering of others.[28] While I am not calling for educators to simply ignore these expressions of suffering and victimization, the priority of these schools should be on instruction and not therapy or politics.

For Bowker, driving the politics and the more general discontent of students is an underlying sense that these institutions are fundamentally dangerous places: "We are primarily concerned with one subset of these demands: the demands set forth by students and protestors that the university undertake significant organizational change because, according to them, the university is a dangerous place" (xvii). This notion of a generalized threat can be traced in part to Left-leaning politics and the concepts of systemic racism, symbolic violence, and an expansive notion of trauma.[29] In fact, for Bowker, university administrators are making things worse by supporting student demands for a protected learning environment:

By forcing the resignation of staff touched by scandal, by shying away from conflict with students or groups who claim to have been victimized in the university, and by failing to defend the boundaries of the university itself, university leaders have colluded with the assumptions underlying protestors' demands and have, ironically, only enlivened conflict and strife on their campuses. What seems to motivate the university to undertake collusive responses when faced with identity-based conflicts is, ironically, a fear of losing control of how it will be known by others and, therefore, of how it will know itself.

(xvi-xvii)

Bowker believes that universities cater to protesting students because they want to control how the institution is perceived by others, but I have argued that many of their responses are driven by a narcissistic desire to be seen as doing the right thing.[30] This need to signal their virtue may be in part related to their repressed acknowledgment of how these schools actually increase inequality and decrease social mobility as they train people to become cynical capitalists competing for rationed resources.[31]

Since elite colleges and universities are obsessed with their rankings, and all colleges grade and rank their students, these institutions are centered on producing winners and losers in a competitive system, but the more that earning grades is privileged over learning, the more students lose their interest in what they are doing: Still many students are still driven to receive the highest reward with the least amount of effort.[32] Of course, no one wants to talk about this dirty underside of education because it is much more comforting to idealize students and the institution. Furthermore, critics – like myself – run the risk of feeding the Right-wing and conservative efforts to defund these schools. However, while Republicans tend to see these colleges and universities as dominated by Leftist seeking to indoctrinate students into a Marxist, communist ideology, I have posited that the bigger threat comes from the devaluing of learning by the privileging of grading.[33]

For Bowker, universities are being undermined by their failure to commit to the values of exploration, experimentation, and self-discovery:

> Whereas the university was once imagined to be a place for exploration, experimentation, identity "moratorium," and self-discovery (see Marcia, 1967; Tobacyk, 1981), it seems to have become a place where individuals with fixed or firmly established identities seek to confirm what they already know to be true about themselves, others, and the world. In this quest for conformation, some elect to do battle with those whose senses of self and other differ from their own.
>
> (xviii)

The idea here is that students no longer desire to learn new things that challenge what they already know; instead, they are focused on having their prior identity affirmed.[34] This type of confirmation bias makes it hard for instructors to challenge their students and expose them to things that are complex, ambiguous, and ambivalent, but we still have to ask where this desire for the same comes from.

As we have seen with the examples of hysteria and narcissism in higher education, young people are searching for meaning and identity, and they often pursue these desires on an unconscious level. Moreover, these quests for a firm sense of self can block learning when education threatens the identities formed through the identification with knowledge.[35] As Lacan argued, just like we defend our bodies against any external threat, we also defend our bodies of knowledge because they help to build our sense of self.[36] In seeing the ego as mainly a defense mechanism, Lacan defines it as the source of repression since people do not want to acknowledge to themselves anything that upsets their previous sense of identity and knowledge.[37] True education then often conflicts with the ego, but Bowker wants to equate the pursuit of knowledge with the development of the autonomous self: "what we "reach for" when we reach "upward" is something akin to the self, variously expressed in such notions as enlightenment, wisdom, and freedom of thought and expression. Reaching upward, then, also means reaching inward, toward an inner spirit or self" (xviii). In equating self-development with the pursuit of knowledge, Bowker may be feeding the mistaken idea that modern reason is centered on free speech and individual freedom.[38] While it is common to see the modern Enlightenment as basing knowledge on freedom, what is really at the center of reason is the ability to distinguish fact from fiction or what Freud called the reality principle.[39] Of course, one has to be free to pursue truth wherever it leads, but that does not mean that modern liberal democracy and science promote individual freedom as the primary objective. There is, thus, a difference between the search for truth and the formation of an identity or self.

Drawing from Winnicott's work, Bowker believes that the goal of university education is to help individual students protect their inner mental life as they carry forward the capacity for creation that can be traced back to their childhood:

> What is at stake in struggles within the university is nothing less than the secu- rity, even the possibility, of an inner world, the defense of which is the defense of the life of the mind, and the defense of the capacity for imaginative con- struction. It is, therefore, the defense of the possibility that the individual can carry forward into adult life something essential about childhood experience: the capacity for creative living, or, in somewhat more oblique language, the capacity "to create the world" (Winnicott, 1986).
>
> (xix)

My fear is that this focus on individual imagination and creativity does not accept the role of reason and universal equality in transcending the individual by replacing the primary processes with the reality principle through the ideals of impartiality and empiricism.[40] In fact, the major reason why universities end up taking on so many different missions, like healing the world and entertaining students, is that they have lost sight of their primary task.[41]

Universities and Reason

Like many other critics of higher education, Bowker feels that a major issue is that universities are treating students like children and not as adults: "At the same time, however, students are treated as children or adolescents. Students are "taken care of" by universities to a great degree, and today's students find themselves catered to by an ever-growing assortment of services and amenities that either imply or state outright that students need and want greater university intervention not only in their educational pursuits but in their personal, professional, and social lives" (xx). Of course, it is often the parents who expect and demand these services, but many students also want to be treated as if they were young children. But once again, we have to ask: Why are the students seeking this care and protection, and why are these schools so willing to provide it?[42]

Bowker is correct to trace some of these issues back to the contradictory ways that students are being represented and treated: "But such efforts make the expe- rience of university life confusing for students, who at one moment are offered countless forms of support and personalized attention, some aimed purely at facilitating their entertainment, and the next moment are accused of belonging to "Generation Me," a uniquely and dangerously "narcissistic" lot, unprepared to survive the harshness of an adult life in which no one will attend to or care about their needs" (xxi-xxii). In this structure, parents over-protect their children, and then they demand that colleges treat them as children, but adults also attack these young people for not being prepared for a harsh reality.[43] Thus, the people who cater to and over-protect students also criticize them for not being responsible adults.

In response to this ambivalent attitude, adults have toward college students, Bowker returns to the notion that educators should not advocate for either side, and instead, they should help these young people discover their true selves: "Rather than align ourselves with or oppose 'some contending party' in university conflicts, we strive to give voice to what Winnicott refers to as the 'true self'" (xxiv). The problem with this solution is that it does not affirm the way that higher education is based on promoting reason and the scientific method, and this form of the reality principle asks people to suspend their self-interest in order to discover the truth of evidence from an unbiased perspective.

Responding to the various ideological conflicts occurring on campus, Bowker insists on something akin to analytic neutrality and the type of impartiality I have discussed previously:

> "Neutrality," in this sense, does not refer to any prohibition against analysts having political convictions and, in the arena of public life, acting on those convictions, but rather against the analyst making statements that might be experienced in the analytic setting as aligning the analyst with the patient's internal objects and the self-judgments associated with identification with those objects. When we speak of replacing judgment with understanding, we have in mind something analogous to analytic neutrality, since we seek to avoid basing our assessment of university conflict on judgments of the moral worth of individuals or groups. Specifically, we do not, by endorsing either a favorable or an unfavorable moral judgment of any group or individual, engage in an act that, however unconsciously, colludes with a defense against powerful unconscious feelings that the self embedded in the group is of little value.
>
> (xxvi)

The problem with this defense of the self in relation to the social group is that universities are supposed to be collective organizations centered on developing universal subjects dedicated to the use of shared, transparent methods in pursuit of the truth.[44] In turning the focus back on the self, there is the risk of catering to a libertarian, individualistic ideology. In this context, the call for neutrality often results in the desire not to critique Right-wing and conservative ideologies.[45]

While I have argued that modern liberal science and democracy are based on an ideology of no ideology, it would be better to say that these two modern institutions rely on the ideals of universality and reason, which is itself defined by the ability to distinguish between truth and fiction.[46] For Bowker, this privileging of equality and reality testing is replaced by a focus on the self: "Translated into the context with which we are concerned here, the implication is that universities should neither impose morally invested ends on students nor offer unquestioning acceptance of the moral judgments students espouse, and that universities, instead, should facilitate internal development in a direction consonant with understanding and self-determination" (xxvii). While Bowker wants higher education to be based on developing the individual agency of students, the goal should be for these young adults to learn how to use reason in order to reach a shared consensus.[47]

The way that psychoanalysis conforms to these modern ideals is that the emphasis on neutrality and reality testing are combined with an overcoming of the pleasure principle and the reliance on unquestioned authority[48]:

> This neutrality is needed because of the way the idea of morality inevitably involves the division of those engaged in conflict into the "good" and the "bad." This division is precisely the goal of the harsh self-assessment to which we have referred, which, by its nature, allows little if any room for nuanced understanding of human motivation beyond that which is organized around good and bad choices driven by good and bad character. Indeed, this "moral orientation" is the expression of the work of harsh internal object relations experienced as a harsh internal self-assessment.
>
> (xxvii)

This presentation of neutrality in psychoanalysis and higher education is problematic because it seeks to call into question all morality, but academic discourse relies on the ethical principles of transparency, honesty, equality, and truth.[49] Moreover, psychoanalysis does not simply suspend morality because this would cater to the individual's pursuit of pleasure; rather, analysis suspends the judgment of the Other so that the subject can freely express their own thoughts and feelings through speech.

Since Bowker wants to emphasize the self, he misrecognizes the shared ideals shaping academic discourse: "The ideal of support for the self stands opposed to the ideal of the university as a moral training ground, devoted to preparing students for their subsequent entry into life in a moral order (on moral order, see Levine, 2017)" (xxvi). Although modernity represented a break with conservative morality, authority, and religion, psychoanalysis is not a libertarian discourse, and the same can be said about higher education.[50] As Freud insisted, in the conflict between social morality and individual liberty, psychoanalysis does not take a side because it recognizes the need to affirm the fundamental human conflict between society and the individual.

Interestingly, Bowker does see that an aspect of college entails the need for individual students to learn how to live with people they do not know: "University living, for many students, means a loss of private space and entry into a world shared with strangers" (5). There is thus a strong collective aspect of higher education, and this exposure to others implies that one learns how to give up the focus on the self in order to affirm a universal mode of subjectivity.[51] Yet, Bowker's dedication to self-psychology blocks his ability to affirm both psychoanalysis and the modern subject of the university:

> The reduction of self to physical being is central to struggles in universities. This reduction makes all that is of value in our personal existence a kind of brute fact about us, something given to us at birth that can never be changed: the self as skin color. In a language used by Christopher Bollas, this reduced self is the self dominated by its "fate," rather than the self as the active moment in pursuit of its "destiny" (1989). In a sense, the struggles in universities over identity are struggles over whether students must submit to their "fate" or can, instead, pursue a "destiny" not predetermined by ascribed or imposed qualities of being, qualities as immutable as those that define their physical existence.
>
> (6)

From this perspective, the major conflict shaping universities and the mental health of their students is the fight between the development of the self and the use of group identity categories, but what I have been arguing is that what students need to learn is how to use reason in order to transcend their own immediate, individual thoughts and feelings. In the goal of having a more just and equal society, everyone should be treated the same as they are taught to pursue a truth that ideally can be accessed by anyone.[52] Just as Descartes argued that the modern scientist has to suspend all bias and self-interest, we need to teach students how to go beyond their isolated selves.[53]

As Bowker rightly indicates, many students who belong to particular identity groups may feel alienated by the push to get them to pursue truth from a universal perspective:

> Claude Steele observes (quoted in Green, 2016) that schools offer black students the opportunity to assimilate into an alien, or white, culture. But, to do so, they must "give up many particulars of being black – styles of speech and appearance," and thereby "learn how little valued they are."
>
> (6–7)

While it is clear that many students do feel alienated in higher education, I would argue that the movement from being a separate self to being part of a universal culture does require a certain level of alienation for everyone.[54] After all, the university is based on universality, and this mode of equality and neutrality requires a submission of the self to reality, truth, and shared, transparent methods.

Instead of catering to individual and group identities and identification, institutions of higher education need to be dedicated to promoting a universal mode of subjectivity. However, for Bowker, one of the reasons why students may feel alienated by this universality is that they are used to judging people based on their social identity:

> The importance of having teachers who "look like" us stems from a construction of the world in which what people look like is the most reliable clue as to

how they think and relate – that is, whether they think and relate like us. If those who look like us also think and relate like us, then being with them places us in a familiar world.

(7)

Due to a mostly Left-wing ideology, educators and students often now think that the defining aspect of education revolves around the individual's affirmation of particular group identities, yet this focus on identity and identification blocks our access to universal subjectivity and modern democratic equality.[55] For Bowker, students want to be taught by teachers who look like them or belong to the same identity group because they feel safer dealing with people who appear familiar, but education should be about learning new things and leaving the safe comfort of always seeing a world that mirrors the self.

Instead of affirming the universal subject of higher education, science, democracy, and psychoanalysis, Bowker emphasizes self-determination as the key to human development:

> But, there is another possibility, which is that the protest against hidden racism, while couched in the language of race, racial identity, and race-based culture, is about something more general, which is the demand for adaptation itself and the resulting loss of self-determination implied in adaptation, no matter what group culture demands the adaptation.
>
> (9)

The problem with this defense of self-determination in higher education is that it blocks the important need to transcend the self through reason and the reality principle.[56] As we have seen, when students spend all of their time focusing on their own thoughts and feelings, they often are prone to being dominated by negative emotions, which leads to anxiety and depression. What students often need to learn is how to escape this self-consciousness by being with others who may be different from themselves while they engage in a mode of thinking that transcends the isolated individual.

In terms of the college mental health crisis, Bowker's desire to stress the role of the self in higher education only serves to heighten the nervous self-consciousness of young adults. Although it looks like psychoanalysis also promotes this type of self-centering, the reality is that through the combination of analytic neutrality and the free association of the patient, what one discovers is that the mind is shaped by an interlocking network of symbolic associations and memories that we never fully control.[57] Furthermore, the way that the reality principle shapes the uncensored discourse of the patient is not by the guidance of an intentional ego; rather, the truth of internal and external reality is assessed through an unintentional flow of a discourse that is not concerned with the self or the Other.[58]

Although it is unrealistic to advocate for every college student to undergo an intensive psychoanalysis, what we can advocate for is a clear articulation of the ideals and principles shaping academic discourse. Not only do we have to help students see the importance of being impartial, but we also have to privilege evidence over pre-suppositions. As Bowker's own work reveals, this need to promote the universal subject of science and democracy is threatened by the reliance on predetermined social identities:

> Proceeding in this way would mean, for example, assigning black students to the victim role because they are black and because all black people are victims, regardless of the particular circumstances of their lives. In other words, it would mean consigning all black people to the role of objects determined by others, rather than subjects determined by themselves.
>
> (18)

While I agree that the acceptance of identities determined by social groups blocks student access to academic discourse, Bowker's solution is also a problem because he returns to the emphasis on the individual's ego. Like many other theorists of education, Bowker's perspective idealizes student agency and fails to see the limits of focusing on the self.[59]

What Bowker does effectively critique is the role of identity politics in higher education, which is often based on a misguided notion of social psychology: "The stronger the identification with an individual or group, the greater the pressure to accept – without question – the interpretation of its condition, an interpretation that holds the group together" (21). From a psychoanalytic perspective, a central problem of group identity is that it often results in suspending critical thinking and reality testing.[60] As Freud showed in his analysis of love, hypnosis, armies, religions, and political rallies, identification with an idealized group relies on the regression of the subject to a position of being a helpless infant who needs to be saved by the Other. Since education relies on critical analysis, this type of tribal identity and thought blocks the foundation of learning and science.

In distinguishing empathy from compassion, Bowker seeks to safeguard the ability of people in a group to understand each other, but this reliance on empathy as an overcoming of group fantasy does not appear to fit the psychoanalytic comprehension of empathic identification: "Unlike compassion, empathy refers to a connection with an individual or group that facilitates movement away from the group's fantasy of itself and toward understanding of the group member's real situation" (21). For Bowker, empathy can help a person understand a group member's reality, but for Freud, empathy is a hysterical identification based on the fantasy of placing the self in the same imagined situation.[61] Unlike the use of empathy in self-psychology, psychoanalysis relies on affirming the radical otherness of the other: On a fundamental level, we never gain direct access to another person's experience or consciousness, but we can agree to commit to the same processes of reason and universal objectivity.[62]

This notion of universality is so important because, as Bowker reports, many students of color feel that others can never know what is feels like to be them: "In response to this interpretation of the Museum's mission, the student insisted that no such communication or understanding was possible, suggesting that the white students and teacher 'cannot understand how it feels to be black'" (22). Instead of trying to cover over this sense of being different, a better strategy may be to affirm radical otherness as one promotes universality as the key to science and democratic equality.[63]

As Bowker indicates, when we do not make reason and objectivity the center of higher education, we end up privileging individual experience: "'Lived experience' has been (conspicuously) spared from modern and postmodern critiques of subjectivity and rationality and, as a result, seems to some to be the only remaining source of cultural authority" (27). In promoting lived personal experience over reason and abstract knowledge, universities undermine their basic principles and often feed individual psychopathologies: "The more we attend to difference (and différance), domination, and the subaltern, the more we mistrust reason and turn to testimonies, embodiments, and other expressions of the lived experiences of the oppressed" (27). As we find in hysteria, once someone claims a victim identity, it becomes difficult to offer any criticism or reality testing.[64] Furthermore, when this type of lived personal experience is challenged, the result is often an aggressive attack on the person who appears to be insensitive to the suffering of the individual. The problem, then, with focusing on trauma, oppression, and victimization in higher education is that it can subvert the ideals of neutrality and reason, but that does not mean that we should simply advocate for an idealized version of history; instead, we have to approach all personal and collective memories by pursuing the truth without fear of upsetting sensitive subjects.

Returning to Trauma in Higher Education

Bowker articulates some of the issues concerning the current desire to see students as traumatized and the need for higher education to protect them against being retraumatized through exposure to discomfiting material:

> Caruth and those trauma theorists who share her views have suggested that we inhabit, or, rather, that we must envision ourselves as inhabiting, a post-traumatic era, a "post-traumatic century" (Felman, 1995, p. 13). One consequence of doing so is that we come to doubt the possibility that historical truth may be preserved in rational thought or expression and, instead, that we turn to fractured testimonies, affects and symptoms, and other artifacts to (re)constitute reality.
>
> (28)

This undermining of historical truth and reason by an emphasis on trauma represents one of the ways that a misunderstanding of psychoanalysis has affected higher education and the college mental health crisis.[65] Since the definition of trauma has been expanded to such an extent, it can be applied to almost everyone and anyone, and as we have seen, when we start seeing our students as traumatized, there is a tendency to try to turn education into therapy. Since trauma is often represented as a personal experience that cannot be symbolized or learned from, it threatens to undermine education and reason.

Bowker correctly criticizes the way that the expansion of the category of trauma has resulted in the absurd claim that history itself is equivalent to the Holocaust:

> We must even approach "his-tory as holocaust" (Felman & Laub, 1992, p. 95), which is to say not that we should attend to this or that holocaust in our study of history, but, rather, that all of history is holocaust, that even our own personal histories may be, in this sense, holocausts, and that to understand what has happened or what is happening to us as individuals and communities, we must put ourselves in the place of one suffering or witnessing a holocaust.
>
> (28)

As I wrote in my book *Teaching the Rhetoric of Resistance*, the focus on a generalized theory of trauma in the humanities often results in losing all sense of proportionality and reason as one idealizes the people who represent themselves as the empathic witnesses to a past traumatic event.[66] Since narcissistic educators want to prove that they are caring, moral people, they are motivated to see their students as victims who can be healed by the teacher's empathy. This misguided model of education and therapy threatens to undermine universities from within.

Bowker points out that this trend to focus on trauma in higher education represents an appeal to unreason and repression of academic principles and modern reason:

> At a minimum, such attitudes would seem to suggest that the reigning view of trauma, experience, and truth is one in which what we think of as reality is not determined by historical accounts, reasons, evidence, or the like, but, rather, by intuitions of terror, apocalyptic imaginations, identifications with victims, and intense emotional reactions.
>
> (28)

Just as Freud saw trauma as causing a repetition of an unsymbolized event, the turn to trauma often entails a privileging of emotion and experience over reason:

> What Benjamin, Caruth, Felman, and others are suggesting, and what has been accepted to a surprising degree in many university cultures, internet cultures, and popular cultures is that, because reality itself is constituted by pervasive yet ultimately unthinkable traumatization, only immediate experiences, memories that 'flash up at a moment of danger,' and visceral identifications with trauma victims lead us to the truth.
>
> (28–29)

In examining the history of trauma studies in the humanities, Bowker identifies the way this emphasis tends to privilege the unthinkable in an institution supposedly centered on thought: One of the sources of our politics of unreason, then, can be found within institutions of higher education.[67]

Although Bowker questions the effects of concentrating on trauma in humanities courses, he also feels that when students ask for trigger warnings and safe spaces, their requests should be respected because if the institution does not affirm these desires, students will identify more with the position of victims confronted with traumatic experiences:

> if the organizations or communities to which they belong seem contemptuous of their requests for help, if requests for care are taken as proof of weakness, cowardice, or other shame-worthy qualities, or if their environments do not seem to be "safe" places to articulate their needs, not least because their expressions of need violate the "freedom" of their teachers. Students who request trigger warnings may experience, in having their requests ridiculed, a form of emotional assault, degradation, and abandonment. Harsh rejections and dismissals of students' expressions of need for protection, then, likely deepen students' vicarious identifications with trauma and with the traumatized.
>
> (32)

It may be hard to prevent this form of empathic identification with trauma and victimization, but one way to try to avoid this issue is to stress the need for emotional distance in relation to cultural material.[68] However, what we are finding instead is that some teachers are bent on making emotional identification the key to education as they cater to the desire of hysterical students to see themselves as victims of culture and history.

As Bowker points out, it is ironic that students want to be protected from being exposed to triggering material in the classroom when they spend so much of their time-consuming cultural material on their own that could be considered threatening:

> These reflections suggest that trigger warnings themselves are not central to the trigger warning debate. That is, merely warning students about the likelihood of encountering explicit material from classrooms would do little to resolve what lies at the heart of students' complaints-since, after all, young people today are exposed to more explicit, violent, and graphic images than perhaps any generation in human history.
>
> (33)

Since there is so much media depicting violent and explicit content being consumed by these students, their call for trigger warnings and safe spaces must stem from a desire to see education as a protective container or substitute family.[69]

In relation to this demand for educational safety, Bowker makes the provocative claim that while schools say that they want to promote diversity, students themselves are afraid of experiencing diverse ideas and content:

> That is, the problem lies not in the fact that the classroom environment is insufficiently diverse so much as that it is excessively diverse: The course group is unsafe because it is not bound by a shared experience and so is unable to reassure its members that their internal reactions will be affirmed by others.
>
> (39)

From the perspective of narcissism, what students really want is to have their thoughts, feelings, and identities affirmed, and this need to treat the world as a reflecting mirror blocks the ability to learn new things about oneself and others.[70]

Bowker argues that a major cause for contemporary student discontent is that they have not developed the internal mental strength to handle the assessments made by others:

> While vulnerability to the words used by others may be inevitable in early emotional development, it does not follow that we must continue, throughout life, to cede power to outside authorities to determine our internal states of mind. On the contrary, the idea of maturation includes the expectation that we will develop internal resources needed to reduce, if not altogether eliminate, our vulnerability to external assessment.
>
> (54)

It is hard to imagine how people can be educated if they cannot tolerate external assessment, but many students today display a strong fear of being judged by others.[71]

Bowker's solution to this problem of students asking to be protected against the ideas and values of others is to call for universities to stop trying to provide moral judgments: "In other words, the university must make a definitive break with the ideal of itself as a moral system that can protect those in it from the dangers posed to them by adverse moral judgment" (66). What I find problematic about this suspension of academic moral judgment is that it does not leave room for the principles of impartiality, universality, honesty, and transparency, which are the ideals of modern liberal science and democracy. As I will argue in the final chapter of this book, there are many things we can do to fix the mental health crisis in higher education, and one key aspect is to define and defend what we mean by the principles of academic discourse. Instead of positing that the modern scientific method is not an ideology and provides no moral guidance, it would be better to promote the principles of impartiality, empiricism, universality, transparency, and honesty.

Notes

1 Bowker, Matthew H., and David P. Levine. *A Dangerous Place to Be: Identity, Conflict, and Trauma in Higher Education*. Routledge, 2018.
2 Levin, Shana, et al. "Ethnic and university identities across the college years: A common in-group identity perspective." *Journal of Social Issues* 65.2 (2009): 287–306.
3 Bronfenbrenner, Urie. "Ecology of the family as a context for human development: Research perspectives." *Adolescents and Their Families* (2013): 1–20.
4 Gavita, Oana Alexandra, Daniel David, and Raymond DiGiuseppe. "You are such a bad child! Appraisals as mechanisms of parental negative and positive affect." *The Journal of general psychology* 141.2 (2014): 113–129.
5 Harter, Susan, et al. "A model of the effects of perceived parent and peer support on adolescent false self behavior." *Child Development* 67.2 (1996): 360–374.
6 Edery, Rivka A. "The traumatic effects of narcissistic parenting on a sensitive child: A case analysis." *Health Science Journal* 13.1 (2019): 1–3.
7 Freud, Sigmund. *On Narcissism: An Introduction*. Read Books Ltd, 2014.
8 Imamoglu, Ahmet, and A. Y. Ş. E. G. Ü. L. Durak Batigün. "The assessment of the relationship between narcissism, perceived parental rearing styles, and defense mechanisms." *Dusunen Adam-Journal of Psychiatry and Neurological Sciences* 33.4 (2020).
9 Lansky, Melvin R. "The 'Incompatible Idea' revisited: The oft-invisible ego-ideal and shame dynamics." *The American Journal of Psychoanalysis* 63 (2003): 365–376.
10 Freud, Sigmund. *Civilization and Its Discontents*. Broadview Press, 2015.
11 Estes, Danielle K. "Managing the student-parent dilemma: Mothers and fathers in higher education." *Symbolic Interaction* 34.2 (2011): 198–219.
12 Maxwell, Claire, Peter Aggleton, and Claudia Lapping. "Institutional accountability and intellectual authority: Unconscious fantasies and fragile identifications in contemporary academic practice." *Privilege, Agency and Affect: Understanding the Production and Effects of Action*. Springer, 2013, 88–105.
13 Casale, Silvia, et al. "Narcissism and authentic self: An unfeasible marriage?" *Personality and Individual Differences* 135 (2018): 131–136.
14 Gerzi, Shmuel. "Trauma, narcissism and the two attractors in trauma." *The International Journal of Psychoanalysis* 86.4 (2005): 1033–1050.
15 Samuels, Robert. *Educating Inequality: Beyond the Political Myths of Higher Education and the Job Market*. Routledge, 2017.
16 Robinson, William I. "Global capitalism and the restructuring of education: The transnational capitalist class' quest to suppress critical thinking." *Social Justice* (2016): 1–24.
17 Collyer, Fran M. "Practices of conformity and resistance in the marketisation of the academy: Bourdieu, professionalism and academic capitalism." *Critical Studies in Education* 56.3 (2015): 315–331.
18 Han, Byung-Chul. *Capitalism and the Death Drive*. John Wiley & Sons, 2021.
19 Hurst, Andrea. "Capitalism and the banality of desire." *Journal of the British Society for Phenomenology* 51.4 (2020): 288–304.
20 Thomas, Jacqueline. *Factors Relating to Student Grade Obsession: A Quantitative Correlational Study*. University of Phoenix, 2011.
21 Cortez, Franz Giuseppe F. "Arithmomanic education and the metric society: The role of the school in the quantification cult." *Kritike* 17.2 (2023): 38.
22 Hageback, Niklas. *The Death Drive: Why Societies Self-Destruct*. Gaudium, 2020.
23 Baumeister, Roy F., and Steven J. Scher. "Self-defeating behavior patterns among normal individuals: Review and analysis of common self-destructive tendencies." *Psychological Bulletin* 104.1 (1988): 3.
24 Sperber, Murray. *Beer and Circus: How Big-Time College Sports Has Crippled Undergraduate Education*. Macmillan, 2000.

25 Armstrong, Elizabeth A., and Laura T. Hamilton. *Paying for the Party: How College Maintains Inequality*. Harvard University Press, 2013.

26 Goldrick-Rab, Sara, and Marshall Steinbaum. "What is the problem with student debt." *Journal of Policy Analysis and Management* 39.2 (2020): 534–540.

27 Spence, Sean A. "Hysteria: A new look." *Psychiatry* 5.2 (2006): 56–60.

28 Shands, Harley C. "How are 'psychosomatic' patients different from 'psychoneurotic' patients?" *Psychotherapy and Psychosomatics* 26.5 (1975): 270–285.

29 Cless, Jessica D., and Briana S. Nelson Goff. "Teaching trauma: A model for introducing traumatic materials in the classroom." *Advances in Social Work* 18.1 (2017): 25–38.

30 Liu, Catherine. *Virtue Hoarders: The Case Against the Professional Managerial Class*. University of Minnesota Press, 2021.

31 Samuels, Robert. "Globalization and its discontents: Revisiting the critique of the centrist global elites." *Psychoanalysis and the Future of Global Politics: Overcoming Climate Change, Pandemics, War, and Poverty*. Cham: Springer Nature Switzerland, 2023, 73–91.

32 Tippin, Gregory K., Kathryn D. Lafreniere, and Stewart Page. "Student perception of academic grading: Personality, academic orientation, and effort." *Active Learning in Higher Education* 13.1 (2012): 51–61.

33 Hancock, Curtis L. "The rhetoric of indoctrination: Cultural Marxist propaganda in American schools." *Człowiek w Kulturze* 31.2 (2021): 4–10.

34 Sherman, David K., et al. "Deflecting the trajectory and changing the narrative: How self-affirmation affects academic performance and motivation under identity threat." *Journal of Personality and Social Psychology* 104.4 (2013): 591.

35 Lee, J. Katherine, Aurelia T. Alston, and Kimberly B. Kahn. "Identity threat in the classroom: Review of women's motivational experiences in the sciences." *Translational Issues in Psychological Science* 1.4 (2015): 321.

36 Lacan, Jacques, Alan Sheridan, and Malcolm Bowie. "Aggressivity in psychoanalysis." *Écrits: A Selection*. Routledge, 2020, 9–32.

37 Muller, John P. "Ego and subject in Lacan." *Psychoanalytic Review* 69.2 (1982): 234.

38 Hayek, Friedrich A. "Freedom, reason, and tradition." *Ethics* 68.4 (1958): 229–245.

39 Samuels, Robert, and Robert Samuels. "Science and the reality principle." *Freud for the Twenty-First Century: The Science of Everyday Life*. Springer, 2019, 5–16.

40 Freud, Sigmund. "Formulations on the two principles of mental functioning." *Standard Edition* 12.1958 (1911): 213–226.

41 Samuels, Robert. *Why Public Higher Education Should Be Free: How to Decrease Cost and Increase Quality at American Universities*. Rutgers University Press, 2019.

42 Perry, Cody J., et al. "Knowledge, use, and perceived value of university student services: International and domestic student perceptions." *Journal of International Students* 10.3 (2020): 613–628.

43 Ungar, Michael. "Overprotective parenting: Helping parents provide children the right amount of risk and responsibility." *The American Journal of Family Therapy* 37.3 (2009): 258–271.

44 Barnett, Ronald. "Recapturing the universal in the university." *Educational Philosophy and Theory* 37.6 (2005): 785–797.

45 Goodman, Kathleen M. "The effects of viewpoint diversity and racial diversity on need for cognition." *Journal of College Student Development* 58.6 (2017): 853–871.

46 Kelly, Paul J. "Impartiality: A philosophical perspective." *Judicial Integrity*. Brill Nijhoff, 2004, 17–42.

47 Leiviskä, Anniina. "Truth, moral rightness, and justification: A Habermasian perspective on decolonizing the university." *Educational Theory* 73.2 (2023): 223–244.

48 Samuels, Robert. "Conclusion: Psychoanalysis and the psychology of global enlightenment." *Psychoanalysis and the Future of Global Politics: Overcoming Climate Change, Pandemics, War, and Poverty*. Cham: Springer Nature Switzerland, 2023, 93–108.

49 Rieff, Philip. *Freud: The Mind of the Moralist*. University of Chicago Press, 1979.

50 Freud, Sigmund. *The Future of an Illusion*. Broadview Press, 2012.
51 Uljens, Michael. "The idea of a universal theory of education – An impossible but necessary project?" *Journal of Philosophy of Education* 36.3 (2002): 353–375.
52 Barry, Brian. *Culture and Equality: An Egalitarian Critique of Multiculturalism*. Harvard University Press, 2002.
53 Descartes, René. "Descartes's discourse on method." *Ratio et Fides: A Preliminary Intro-duction to Philosophy for Theology*. Wipf and Stock Publishers, 2018, 109.
54 Blunden, Andy. "The subjective notion: Universal, individual and particular." *Hegel for Social Movements*. Brill, 2019, 115–127.
55 Gitlin, Todd. "The rise of 'identity politics': An examination and a critique." *Higher Education Under Fire*. Routledge, 2020, 308–325.
56 Hartmann, Heinz. "Notes on the reality principle." *The Psychoanalytic Study of the Child* 11.1 (1956): 31–53.
57 Leavy, Stanley A. "Self and sign in free association." *The Psychoanalytic Quarterly* 62.3 (1993): 400–421.
58 Barratt, Barnaby B. "Opening to the otherwise: The discipline of listening and the necessity of free-association for psychoanalytic praxis." *The International Journal of Psychoanalysis* 98.1 (2017): 39–53.
59 Wright, Gloria Brown. "Student-centered learning in higher education." *International Journal of Teaching and Learning in Higher Education* 23.1 (2011): 92–97.
60 Freud, Sigmund. *Group Psychology and the Analysis of the Ego*. WW Norton & Company, 1975.
61 Samuels, Robert. "Populism as a cultural virus." *Viral Rhetoric: Psychoanalysis, Philosophy, and Politics after Covid-19*. Cham: Springer International Publishing, 2021, 79–92.
62 Laplanche, Jean. *Essays on Otherness*. Psychology Press, 1999.
63 Leiviskä, Anniina. "The issue of 'radical otherness' in contemporary theories of democracy and citizenship education." *Journal of Philosophy of Education* 52.3 (2018): 498–514.
64 Samuels, Robert, and Robert Samuels. "Pathos, Hysteria, and the left." *Zizek and the Rhetorical Unconscious: Global Politics, Philosophy, and Subjectivity*. Springer, 2020, 33–47.
65 Kirmayer, Laurence J., Joseph P. Gone, and Joshua Moses. "Rethinking historical trauma." *Transcultural Psychiatry* 51.3 (2014): 299–319.
66 Samuels, Robert. *Teaching the Rhetoric of Resistance: The Popular Holocaust and Social Change in a Post-9/11 World*. Springer, 2007.
67 Rensmann, Lars. *The Politics of Unreason: The Frankfurt School and the Origins of Modern Antisemitism*. Suny Press, 2017.
68 Pihlström, Sami, and Sari Kivistö. *Critical Distance: Ethical and Literary Engagements with Detachment, Isolation, and Otherness*. Springer, 2023.
69 Lukianoff, Greg, and Jonathan Haidt. *The Coddling of the American Mind: How Good Intentions and Bad Ideas Are Setting Up a Generation for Failure*. Penguin, 2019.
70 Howes, Satoris S., et al. "When and why narcissists exhibit greater hindsight bias and less perceived learning." *Journal of Management* 46.8 (2020): 1498–1528.
71 Marinho, Anna Carolina Ferreira, et al. "Fear of public speaking: Perception of college students and correlates." *Journal of Voice* 31.1 (2017): 127.e7.

Chapter 8

Fixing the College Mental Health Crisis

Throughout this book, I have documented several different causes for what is being perceived to be a mental health crisis on college campuses.[1] Some of the sources for student suffering and complaints can be derived from the way parents are now treating their children. For instance, we have seen how a general shift from paternal authority to maternal care has resulted in young people expecting their caregivers to recognize and affirm their symptoms and their displays of competence.[2] In turn, educational institutions train these young people to compete for scarce resources (grades), but this focus on earning undermines their interest in learning.[3] We also have witnessed how social media technologies can become addictive and isolating, and they can also feed a hysterical identification and victim complex.[4] As a way of gaining a stable identity, young adults turn to sites like TikTok to affirm a diagnostic identity and to share the suffering of others.[5] Furthermore, since many students come to campus with prescribed medication and a diagnosis derived from the standard diagnostic manual (DSM), they believe that it is the college's responsibility to take care of their mental health issues.[6]

When these schools become overwhelmed by the number of students with mental health issues, they often rely on ineffective forms of therapy, which I have shown are in part based on the repression of psychoanalysis. Since these institutions want to be seen as being good and caring, they affirm the students' suffering without looking at the deeper causes of their complaints. Meanwhile, many teachers are engaging in what is now called trauma-informed pedagogy because they believe that most or all students suffer from PTSD, and the causes for this trauma range from actual abuse to growing up in an unequal world threatened by climate change.[7] In order to deal with this perceived traumatization, some teachers take on the position of being therapists – even though they have no training to perform this social function.[8]

Colleges and universities are now spending huge amounts of money on accommodating students with mental health issues, and this spending can draw funds away from the core educational mission.[9] In fact, as we have seen, the focus on student emotions can undermine the modern academic emphasis on reason and the scientific method. Thus, the first thing to do in order to combat this mental health crisis is to define and defend the core principles of modern science and democracy.

DOI: 10.4324/9781003545668-8

On the most basic level, we need to teach students that they are being trained and assessed on their ability to use shared methods to discover the truth through the impartial analysis of empirical evidence. As Descartes argued, this need to be impartial not only shapes the modern scientific method but also defines democratic law as based on the neutrality of the judge and jury coupled with the equal treatment of all people.[10]

Universities and colleges have lost sight of these core modern values because these institutions have taken on many different functions – like providing students with mental health counseling and classroom therapy. There is also the issue of teachers using their classes as a substitute form of political activism, and many students now desire for their courses to be centered on particular political ideologies.[11] In response to this politicization of these schools, I have called for them to stop inviting external and internal speakers to talk about politics and other divisive issues. To do this, it might take defunding the programs and groups that support the importing of controversial figures.[12] While students and faculty should be allowed to voice their political opinions on their own time, the classroom should be a place dedicated to facts and not opinions.[13]

Another clear solution, which will be difficult to implement, is to eliminate the use of all phones and laptops in the classroom.[14] It is clear that these devices alienate and distract students, and there is no way to control the addictive use of these media technologies unless one simply bans them from being used during class.[15] I have found that many students are actually thankful for being forced to take a break from their obsessive employment of these devices. Not only does it help their attention to the class material, but it also can push them to participate more in class discussions.[16] Although some teachers argue that they do not want to police their students, it is still necessary to set some limits. In fact, if we start to see media use as a mode of addiction, we will be better able to at least stop this form of escape and self-medication in the classroom.[17]

When teachers say that they do not want to police their students, one of the things they are revealing is that contemporary society has moved away from resolving what Freud called the Oedipus complex. While most people equate this complex with wanting to have sex with the mother and desiring to kill off the interfering father, on a more symbolic level, the Oedipus complex reveals how human drives are shaped by the pleasure principle and the compulsion to pursue the production and release of stimulation without any interference or regulation.[18] Just as addictions can be self-destructive and anti-social, the compulsive use of media technologies feeds a borderline mode of psychopathology.[19] Since the enjoying subject wants to resist any external efforts to limit access to pleasure, a libertarian ideology results from this pursuit of pleasure.[20]

In response to the student's compulsive drives, many institutions simply cater to them because they do not want to be seen as playing the role of the intervening authority. Since patriarchy has been demonized by an emphasis on maternal care, there is no way of pushing people to replace their ego-driven ids with respect for limitations and delay.[21] Although I do not think the solution is to return to the conservative ideology of patriarchal authority, it is still necessary to impose some form of structure and regulation. However, as I have depicted, a misguided notion of psychotherapy has motivated people to see the role of parents, teachers, and administrators as being defined by empathy and affirmation. As part of the self-esteem movement and positive psychology, the role of parents and other adults in relation to young people has been reshaped, and in many cases, what we find is that narcissistic adults are catering to the demands of young people because these adults want to be seen as being virtuous.[22] As Lacan highlighted, underlying the desire to be seen as being good is an unconscious sense of shame that is covered over by having the good self recognized by others.[23]

Lacan also argued that behind every demand for an object, there is a desire for unconditional love, recognition, and knowledge.[24] Drawing from Freud's theory of crying babies, Lacan found that at an early age, children learn that when they display their suffering, caregivers will respond by recognizing their pain and under-standing what they need to do in order to make the suffering go away.[25] As the essence of the transference demands, people want to be saved by others, but for the obsessional narcissist, they want this ideal Other only to affirm their thoughts and feelings, and so the Other becomes neutralized. Perhaps Lacan's biggest contribu-tion to analysis is that he realized that the analyst must find a way to remain neu-tral while still not feeding this desire for an Other who only affirms the subject.[26] Lacan developed several techniques, like making interpretations that were equivo-cal, in order to upset the narcissistic and hysterical desire for love, recognition, and knowledge from a person who has no will of their own.[27]

In terms of education, we also want teachers to be neutral and impartial, but we also do not want them simply to affirm the ideas and feelings of their students. Unfortunately, many instructors now feel that the key to social justice and educa-tion is empathy, but this notion of identifying with the suffering of others often acts to reinforce the hysterical victim complex.[28] As I have articulated throughout this book, what most people do not understand or accept about hysteria is that it is based on the use of suffering in order to gain a stable identity as one manipulates others on an unconscious basis. Of course, many people hate this idea because it looks like blaming the victim, but what we learn from psychoanalysis is that the main issue is how people use their own real and imagined suffering and how this expres-sion of pain produces what Freud called the "secondary gain."[29] On a fundamental level, since it is wrong to criticize the victim, the subject is able to gain a sense of moral purity, while all forms of aggressive vengeance are justified.[30] By splitting the world between a good self and an evil other, a polarized worldview is created, and this type of mentality avoids all ambiguity, complexity, and ambivalence.[31]

When teachers affirm that all of their students are victims of trauma, they cater to this mode of hysteria, which functions to block education and critical thinking. In fact, some instructors refuse to grade their students because they see grading as a form of symbolic violence that retraumatizes students.[32] One of the problems of this educational approach is that it undermines our ability to test reality and accu-rately assess the student's level of knowledge and skill.[33] In other words, the focus on emotions and trauma undermines the foundations of the modern meritocracy, and while there are good reasons to critique this ideology, the basic driving idea is that a society based on inherited social hierarchy (aristocracy) should be replaced by one centered on accurate assessment of knowledge and skill.[34] Even though people with money and power can corrupt this ideal, it is still necessary for institutions to play this function of judgment and credentialing.[35]

Against the ideals of meritocracy, many activists on the Left say that in an unequal society, it is unfair to judge everyone by the same criteria.[36] In other words, the notion of universal judgment and equal treatment is replaced by an emphasis on equity. However, we have to ask the proponents of this Left-leaning ideology what happens when individual teachers try to judge the level of inequity facing particular students or specific identity groups. Instead of trying to make sure that our societies are as equal and fair as possible, the result is to provide special accommodations, and this stress on particularity undermines the universality of the university.

As important modern social institutions, universities and colleges should be dedicated to producing universal subjects that take an unbiased perspective on empirical evidence in order to discover and communicate the truth of reality.[37] This universality also shapes the ideals of a meritocracy because we want to trust that our schools are accurately testing students according to the same shared standards.[38] After all, do we want the person performing brain surgery on us to have gained their position based on the fact that they were promoted in school because of their special circumstances? Many people hate this question, and they argue that if we really stuck to a pure meritocracy, certain social groups would be under-represented in important fields, but the way to deal with this issue is to make society as a whole more just and fair.[39] When universities start believing their mission is to fix all social problems, they lose sight of their core mission of instruction and research.

Although I am promoting the ideals of the modern educational meritocracy, there remains the issue of what to do about the way students have been socialized only to care about their grades and not what they are learning.[40] I have argued that this type of educational structure breeds borderline subjects pursuing their own rewards at any cost, and this type of anti-social mentality leads to cheating and other forms of dishonesty.[41] The first way to respond to this problem is to insist on a fair and transparent mode of assessment and to resist any requests for special treatment. However, since society today often presents a college degree as the only path to success and a good life, we have to find ways to separate grading and learning as much as possible. Once again, a part of the solution is to teach the principles of impartiality, reality testing, universality, and equality. As Freud insisted, we have to find a way to replace the pleasure principle with the reality principle, and part of this process requires delaying immediate pleasure.[42] In terms of education, one possible method to separate pleasure from reason is to start off courses with many ungraded assignments, but eventually, students need to be assessed by using shared standards.[43]

Higher Education Politics

To make higher education more effective and equal, we have to insist on the ideals of modern liberal democracy and science, but as we have seen, these ideals have been challenged by several different political ideologies. From the perspective of many conservatives and people on the Right, higher education has been taken over by a covert Marxist plot to convert students into anti-American communists.[44] As a way of responding to the perceived growing power of women and people of color in society, a political effort has been made to demonize courses and majors that pay special attention to minoritized subjects.[45] As part of the reaction to affirmative action policies, Republicans tend to attack Diversity, Equity, and Inclusion programs in order to protect what they see as the threats being made to white Christian males.[46] We have also seen a strong promotion of academic freedom when it suits their purposes, which is often an indirect call for more conservative and Right-wing faculty and speakers.[47] In their promotion of what they call the diversity of viewpoints, they criticize what has now been called cancel culture and political correctness.[48]

As I have argued, from the perspective of science and universal reason, it makes no sense for universities to promote diverse ideologies since the goal is to affirm the ideology of modern science, which is itself structured by the ideals of impartiality and empiricism.[49] By calling for different ideologies to be aired on an equal basis, one might think that one is promoting the pursuit of truth, but the reality is that combining together two extreme distortions of reality does not help one to discover empirical facts. Too many people then confuse free speech with academic freedom, and what should be valorized is the pursuit of truth wherever it leads and not the ability of everyone to have their opinions voiced.

On a fundamental level, the Republican attack on higher education is mostly a recruiting tool used to demonize Democrats.[50] Since liberals and the Left are often associated with higher education, one way to rally conservative and Right-wing voters is to present examples of extreme Left-wing practices at universities and colleges.[51] Although it should be easy to show that the attacks by the Republicans are based on pure exaggeration and paranoia, the truth is that many of the things they attack are actually happening, but probably not to the degree that is claimed.[52] In fact, we have seen that some teachers do not want to grade students because they see assessment as a form of symbolic violence and discrimination.[53] We have also encountered faculty who feel that every student has been traumatized by systemic racism and inequality, and so the goal of education is to either change the world or to heal the student, who is now represented as being a victim of the dominant society.

In response to some of the more extreme rhetoric coming from the Left, centrist administrators often cater to irrational ideas because they want to be seen as being good people.[54] Thus, an entire institution can be shaped by the narcissistic need to have the ideal self recognized by others. Moreover, I have argued that Freud's theory of hysteria can help us to understand some of the Leftist protests and student discontent because what we find behind these displays of suffering is a desire to be recognized by others, while social authority is seen as being a form of symbolic violence.[55] In catering to student hysteria from the position of narcissism, the quest to base education on reason and equality is undermined.

One possible solution to this problem is to separate education from politics, therapy, and parenting clearly. In other words, schools have to make an effort not to take on different social roles – even when students and parents want them to perform these other functions.[56] Universities and colleges could reduce their spending and enhance their instruction if they re-dedicated themselves to the modern principles of science and democracy.[57] Although science is not determined by democratic voting, modern science and democracy share the same desire for a universal subject.[58] In saying that the subject of democracy is universal, I mean that everyone should be treated equally by the law, and every person's vote should count on an equal basis. Also, ideally, public policy would be based on empirical testing and not ideology, and in this way, democracy relies on science.[59] Democracies also need citizens who can test reality and not be taken in by conspiracy theories and fake forms of information.[60] When we claim that we teach students to be critical thinkers, we mean that we promote the liberal ideals of the reality principle, which requires introspection from a neutral perspective.[61]

While there really is no true liberal party in the United States, many false forms of liberalism are presented. For instance, many popular podcasters and YouTubers claim that they also resist the ideologies of the Left and the Right and are basing their views on a rational perception of the evidence. However, many of these entertainers are really libertarians who demonize the Left and see universities as hotbeds of political correctness and cancel culture.[62] Since these mostly-men like to hear themselves speak for hours without interruption, they are against anything that threatens their free speech.[63] Many of these libertarian entertainers are comedians, like Joe Rogan and Bill Maher, who attack trigger warnings and safe spaces because they want to have the ability to say offensive things to produce the laughter of their audience.[64] Yet, as Freud found in his analysis of jokes, a key aspect of comedy is that it turns suffering into pleasure and the serious into the unserious as it suspends all criticisms.[65] In this model of entertainment, we see how the pleasure principle is able to overcome the reality principle by placing social content in a context where it cannot be analyzed through reason.

Since so many students gain information about the world through entertainment, they have become addicted to a mode of enjoyment that undermines the foundations of education.[66] As Neil Postman described in his *Amusing Ourselves to Death*, entertainment has infected all aspects of our culture – including journalism, politics, and education, and the result is that we have found an easy escape from dealing with reality.[67] For students growing up in this culture, it is not easy to sit in a class and listen to a teacher speak or to spend time dealing with other students while trying to use reason to discover the truth about internal and external reality.[68]

I have argued that psychoanalysis offers the most effective theory and treatment for this culture, but it has been repressed because people do not see it as being scientific or efficient.[69] Instead of relying on Freud, universities often turn to a biological model of human subjectivity that caters to a pharmaceutical solution to human suffering. Even though many of the claims coming from neuroscience and evolutionary psychology can never be fully proven, these fields feed off a perverse incentive system that privileges the biological, medical model of the human mind.[70]

When students are not being told that medication is the solution to their mental disorders, they are often sent to some form of CBT, which I have described as a repackaged mode of hypnotic suggestion.[71] Instead of allowing people to explore the causes and reasons for their mental suffering, they are trained on how to replace bad thoughts and feelings with good ones. While some people with certain limited phobias and obsessions can be helped in the short term by CBT, for the most part, this form of therapy does nothing for them in the long run.[72]

In confusing minds with brains and humans with other animals and computers, our understanding of consciousness, free will, pleasure, and reason is greatly diminished; meanwhile, psychoanalytic theories are rejected because they are said to lack a scientific basis, but I have shown that psychoanalysis is a true science because it provides an impartial view of human experience and thought as it applies reason and reality testing to our inner experiences and external behaviors. Although it is hard to imagine psychoanalysis being used on a wide-scale basis in higher education, it could be applied before people enter college. Moreover, we need to use psychoanalytic theory to understand narcissism, hysteria, and addiction, yet it seems that the more these theories and practices are needed, the less they are respected and used. I hope this book offers a step in the right direction by employing psychoanalysis to fix the college mental health crisis.

Notes

1 Kadison, Richard, and Theresa Foy DiGeronimo. *College of the Overwhelmed: The Campus Mental Health Crisis and What to Do about It*. Vol. 6. San Francisco, CA: Jossey-Bass, 2004.
2 Zakeri, Hamidreza, and Maryam Karimpour. "Parenting styles and self-esteem." *Procedia-Social and Behavioral Sciences* 29 (2011): 758–761.
3 Samuels, Robert. *Educating Inequality: Beyond the Political Myths of Higher Education and the Job Market*. Routledge, 2017.
4 Hull, Mariam, and Mered Parnes. "Tics and TikTok: Functional tics spread through social media." *Movement Disorders Clinical Practice* 8.8 (2021): 1248–1252.
5 Nagy, Péter, et al. "TikTok and tics: The possible role of social media in the exacerbation of tics during the COVID lockdown." *Ideggyogyaszati Szemle/Clinical Neuroscience* 75.5–6 (2022): 211–216.
6 Carter, Gertrude C., and Jeffrey S. Winseman. "Increasing numbers of students arrive on college campuses on psychiatric medications: Are they mentally ill?" *Journal of College Student Psychotherapy* 18.1 (2003): 3–10.
7 Brunzell, Tom, Helen Stokes, and Lea Waters. "Shifting teacher practice in trauma-affected classrooms: Practice pedagogy strategies within a trauma-informed positive education model." *School Mental Health* 11.3 (2019): 600–614.
8 Harrison, Neil, Jacqueline Burke, and Ivan Clarke. "Risky teaching: Developing a trauma-informed pedagogy for higher education." *Teaching in Higher Education* 28.1 (2023): 180–194.

9 Cornish, Peter A., et al. "Meeting the mental health needs of today's college student: Reinventing services through Stepped Care 2.0." *Psychological services* 14.4 (2017): 428.

10 Descartes, René. "Descartes's discourse on method." *Ratio et Fides: A Preliminary Intro-Duction to Philosophy for Theology.* Wipf and Stock Publishers, 2018, 109.

11 Hytten, Kathy. "Teaching as and for activism: Challenges and possibilities." *Philosophy of Education* 2014 (2017): 385–394.

12 Goldberg, Suzanne B. "Free expression on campus: Mitigating the costs of contentious speakers." *Harvard Journal of Law & Public Policy* 41 (2018): 163.

13 Fish, Stanley. *Save the World on Your Own Time.* Oxford University Press, 2008.

14 Selwyn, Neil, and Jesper Aagaard. "Banning mobile phones from classrooms – An opportunity to advance understandings of technology addiction, distraction and cyberbullying." *British Journal of Educational Technology* 52.1 (2021): 8–19.

15 Yamamoto, Kevin. "Banning laptops in the classroom: Is it worth the hassles?" *Journal of Legal Education* 57.4 (2007): 477–520.

16 Jackson, Lorraine D. "Is mobile technology in the classroom a helpful tool or a distraction?: A report of university students' attitudes, usage practices, and suggestions for policies." *International Journal of Technology, Knowledge and Society* 8.5 (2013): 129.

17 Al-Barashdi, Hafidha, Abdelmajid Bouazza, and Naeema Jabur. "Smartphone addiction among university undergraduates: A literature review." *Journal of Scientific Research and Reports* 4.3 (2015): 210–225.

18 Samuels, Robert, and Robert Samuels. "Catharsis: The politics of enjoyment." *Zizek and the Rhetorical Unconscious: Global Politics, Philosophy, and Subjectivity.* Springer, 2020, 7–31.

19 Kienast, Thorsten, et al. "Borderline personality disorder and comorbid addiction: Epidemiology and treatment." *Deutsches Ärzteblatt International* 111.16 (2014): 280.

20 Dervin, Dan. "Political leaders and psychohistorical approaches in a time of borderline polarization." *Journal of Psychohistory* 43.2 (2015).

21 Smith, Joseph C., and Carla J. Ferstman. *The Castration of Oedipus: Feminism, Psychoanalysis, and the Will to Power.* NYU Press, 1996.

22 Heaven, Patrick, and Joseph Ciarrochi. "Parental styles, gender and the development of hope and self-esteem." *European Journal of Personality: Published for the European Association of Personality Psychology* 22.8 (2008): 707–724.

23 Vanheule, Stijn. "Caring and its impossibilities – A Lacanian perspective." *Organisational and Social Dynamics* 2.2 (2002): 264–284.

24 Ahmadzadeh, Shideh. "The study of desire: A Lacanian perspective." *Teaching English Language* 1.2 (2007): 139–153.

25 Samuels, Robert. "Freud's project." *(Mis) Understanding Freud with Lacan, Zizek, and Neuroscience.* Cham: Springer International Publishing, 2022, 7–28.

26 Rabinovich, Diana. "What is a Lacanian clinic?" *The Cambridge Companion to Lacan* (2003): 208–220.

27 Ouvry, Olivier. "Interpretation and equivocation." *Research in Psychoanalysis* 1 (2018): 66–73.

28 Segal, Elizabeth A., and M. Alex Wagaman. "Social empathy as a framework for teaching social justice." *Journal of Social Work Education* 53.2 (2017): 201–211.

29 Freud, Sigmund. *Dora: An Analysis of a Case of Hysteria.* Simon and Schuster, 1997.

30 Cole, Alyson Manda. *The Cult of True Victimhood: From the War on Welfare to the War on Terror.* Stanford University Press, 2007.

31 Schulz, Clarence G. "The struggle toward ambivalence." *Psychiatry* 47.1 (1984): 28–36.

32 Santos, Marc C. "How I implemented Asao B. Inoue's labor-based grading and other antiracist assessment strategies." *CEA Critic* 84.2 (2022): 160–179.

33 Samuels, Robert. *Teaching Writing, Rhetoric, and Reason at the Globalizing University.* Routledge, 2020.

34 Daniels, Norman. "Merit and meritocracy." *Philosophy & Public Affairs* (1978): 206–223.

35 Mijs, Jonathan J. B. "The unfulfillable promise of meritocracy: Three lessons and their implications for justice in education." *Social Justice Research* 29 (2016): 14–34.

36 Sandel, Michael J. "How meritocracy fuels inequality – part II reply to critics." *American Journal of Law and Equality* 1 (2021): 146–166.

37 Barnett, Ronald. "Recapturing the universal in the university." *Educational Philosophy and Theory* 37.6 (2005): 785–797.

38 Bills, David B. "The problem of meritocracy: The belief in achievement, credentials and justice." *Research Handbook on the Sociology of Education*. Edward Elgar Publishing, 2019, 88–105.

39 Liu, Amy. "Unraveling the myth of meritocracy within the context of US higher education." *Higher Education* 62 (2011): 383–397.

40 Thomas, Jacqueline. *Factors Relating to Student Grade Obsession: A Quantitative Correlational Study*. University of Phoenix, 2011.

41 Nyamasvisva, Elisha Tadiwa, et al. "Prevalence of premeditated academic dishonesty at university level. A case study." *Age* 21.24 (2020): 64–68.

42 Freud, Sigmund. "Formulations on the two principles of mental functioning." *Standard Edition* 12.1958 (1911): 213–226.

43 Freud, Sigmund. "Formulations on the two principles of mental functioning." *Standard Edition* 12.1958 (1911): 213–226.

44 Cruz, Ted. *Unwoke: How to Defeat Cultural Marxism in America*. Simon and Schuster, 2023.

45 Rufo, Christopher F. "DEI cult; The University of South Florida turns left-wing racialism into a psychological conditioning program." *City Journal* (2023): NA–NA.

46 Dryden, Joe. "Protecting diverse thought in the free marketplace of ideas: Conservatism and free speech in higher education." *Texas Review of Law & Politics* 23 (2018): 229.

47 Parker, Kim. "The growing partisan divide in views of higher education." *Pew Research Center* 19 (2019).

48 Lukianoff, Greg, and Rikki Schlott. *The Canceling of the American Mind: Cancel Culture Undermines Trust and Threatens Us All – But There Is a Solution*. Simon and Schuster, 2023.

49 Anderson, Charles W. *Prescribing the Life of the Mind: An Essay on the Purpose of the University, the Aims of Liberal Education, the Competence of Citizens, and the Cultivation of Practical Reason*. University of Wisconsin Press, 1993.

50 Giroux, Henry A. "Higher education under siege: Implications for public intellectuals." *Thought & Action* 22.2 (2006): 63–78.

51 Ruth, Jennifer, Valerie C. Johnson, and Ellen Schrecker, eds. *The Right to Learn: Resisting the Right-Wing Attack on Academic Freedom*. Beacon Press, 2024.

52 Wilson, John K. *The Myth of Political Correctness: The Conservative Attack on Higher Education*. Duke University Press, 2020.

53 Inoue, Asao B. *Antiracist Writing Assessment Ecologies: Teaching and Assessing Writing for a Socially Just Future*. Parlor Press LLC, 2015.

54 Kumari, Dimuthu, and R. L. S. Fernando. "Determinants of student activism in state universities in Sri Lanka." *International Journal of Social Science and Human Research* 5.2 (2022): 583–725.

55 Samuels, Robert, and Robert Samuels. "Pathos, Hysteria, and the left." *Zizek and the Rhetorical Unconscious: Global Politics, Philosophy, and Subjectivity*. Springer, 2020, 33–47.

56 Kerr, Clark. "The multiversity." *City of Intellect: The Uses and Abuses of the University*, Cambridge University Press, 2023, 253.

57 Samuels, Robert. *Why Public Higher Education Should Be Free: How to Decrease Cost and Increase Quality at American Universities*. Rutgers University Press, 2019.

58 Casanova, Pablo González. "Universal democracy and the social sciences." *Current Sociology* 46.2 (1998): 29–38.

59 Smith, Kevin B., and Christopher Larimer. *The Public Policy Theory Primer.* Routledge, 2018.

60 Moore, Alfred. "Conspiracies, conspiracy theories and democracy." *Political Studies Review* 16.1 (2018): 2–12.

61 Samuels, Robert, and Robert Samuels. "Science and the reality principle." *Freud for the Twenty-First Century: The Science of Everyday Life.* Springer, 2019, 5–16.

62 Dowling, David O., Patrick R. Johnson, and Brian Ekdale. "Hijacking journalism: Legitimacy and metajournalistic discourse in right-wing podcasts." *Media and Communication* 10.3 (2022): 17–27.

63 Franks, Mary Anne. "The lost cause of free speech." *Journal of Free Speech Law* 2 (2022): 337.

64 Johansson, Christer. "YouTube podcasting, the new orality, and diversity of thought: intermediality, media history, and communication theory as methodological approaches." *Digital Human Sciences: New Objects-New Approaches*, Stockhom University Press, 2021, 253–284.

65 Freud, Sigmund. *The Joke and Its Relation to the Unconscious.* Penguin, 2003.

66 Winzer, Donald L. *Are You Kidding Me? Comparing Student Perceptions and Recall of Comedy and Hard News.* Diss. Indiana University of Pennsylvania, 2019.

67 Postman, Neil. *Amusing Ourselves to Death: Public Discourse in the Age of Show Business.* Penguin, 2005.

68 Samuels, Robert. *Generation X and the Rise of the Entertainment Subject.* Rowman & Littlefield, 2021.

69 Petocz, Agnes. "The scientific status of psychoanalysis revisited." *Philosophy, Science, and Psychoanalysis.* Routledge, 2018, 145–277.

70 Samuels, Robert, and Robert Samuels. "Drugging discontent: Psychoanalysis, drives, and the governmental university medical pharmaceutical complex (GUMP)." *Psychoanalyzing the Politics of the New Brain Sciences.* Springer, 2017, 115–136.

71 Golden, William L. "Cognitive-behavioral hypnotherapy for anxiety disorders." *Journal of Cognitive Psychotherapy* 8.4 (1994): 265.

72 Nadiga, Deepa N., Paula L. Hensley, and E. H. Uhlenhuth. "Review of the long-term effectiveness of cognitive behavioral therapy compared to medications in panic disorder." *Depression and Anxiety* 17.2 (2003): 58–64.

Index